PARTNERS IN CHANGE

Rose Echlin

with additional material from Judith Buck

Published by the King's Fund Centre
126 Albert Street
London
NW1 7NF
Tel: 0171-267 6111

ISBN 1 85717 085 7

A CIP catalogue record for this book is available from the British Library

Distributed by Bournemouth English Book Centre (BEBC)
PO Box 1496
Poole
Dorset
BH12 3YD

The King's Fund Centre is a service development agency which promotes improvements in health and social care. We do this by working with people in health and social services, in voluntary agencies, and with the users of these services. We encourage people to try out new ideas, provide financial or practical support to new developments, and enable experiences to be shared through workshops, conferences, information services and publications. Our aim is to ensure that good developments in health and social care are widely taken up. The King's Fund Centre is part of the King's Fund.

Contents

Preface

Better Futures was a two-year project which focused on improving the quality of life of people with serious and long-term mental health problems. During the period 1992-4, the King's Fund Centre funded a programme of development work in five localities in England and Wales – Clwyd, Leeds, Salford, Swindon and Tower Hamlets. Working in partnership with service users, carers, statutory and voluntary agencies, each locality developed its own programme of work based on local need, context and service provision. The project has produced a variety of ongoing service developments.

The major areas of work were:

- service user participation – helping service users to speak for themselves;
- individual care planning – helping professionals to identify and apply good practice;
- needs-led services – using small grants to set up individualised services, such as a community artist post, and a work introduction scheme;
- planning a community mental health service. In one locality, the work involved the reprovision of acute services from the local psychiatric hospital and the development of a pilot local mental health service.

The ideas in this booklet come mainly from reports on the action learning programmes carried out during 1993-4 in three of the project localities – Clwyd, Leeds and Swindon – which focused on assessment and care planning for individual service users, and from discussions of a working group which met at the King's Fund Centre during 1994. The members of the working group were Thurstine Basset, Jim Brooks, Judith Buck, Rose Echlin, Sara Hammond-Rowley, Veronica Hilton and Barry Wood. The initial reports were written by Thurstine Basset (Swindon), Roger Blunden (Clwyd) and Judith Buck and Rose Echlin (Leeds).

Names and identifying details of both service users and workers in our examples have been changed to protect individual privacy. As far as possible, all the material has been checked out with the people concerned.

Partners in Change will be of primary interest to mental health workers in health and social services and their managers. These will include workers in acute and long-term community mental health teams as well as in day and residential services in both statutory and voluntary sectors. Our work will also be of interest to primary care staff who provide continuing care to mental health service users. We have also attempted to draw out the implications of good care planning for health and social services commissioners.

Acknowledgements

Thanks are particularly due to:

- the service users who contributed their time and experiences to this work. Without them, *Partners in Change* could not have happened;
- the members of the action learning groups in Clwyd, Leeds and Swindon who made time for the work in their already hectic schedules and contributed their ideas, experiences and written material to this booklet;
- Thurstine Basset, Jim Brooks, Judith Buck, Sara Hammond-Rowley, Veronica Hilton, and Barry Wood who took part in a working group which met at the King's Fund Centre during 1994 and drew together the lessons from the three local projects;
- Margaret Hirst, Joan Tugwell and Andrew Wilcox-Jones who contributed some of the written material;
- Janet Hadley who edited the original manuscript.

Chapter 1

Beyond the rhetoric

The lives of many people who have serious and enduring mental health problems can be dominated by dull routine, isolation and hopelessness. For most, there are few opportunities for exercising the choice and control which could lead to real improvements in their quality of life. Changes in this situation can be brought about by professionals supporting service users to achieve the goals that they themselves identify as being important for a better life.

Partnerships with professionals and service users working together to bring about change in people's lives can evolve in the process of individual needs assessment and care planning. Better Futures projects have explored the nature of effective partnerships and have demonstrated how people's lives can be changed for the better. They have done so against a background of considerable change and confusion within the community care system.

The Care Programme Approach (CPA) and Care Management have been introduced, if not fully applied, in the health service and local authorities. Recently, supervision registers have made their appearance. There is a real danger that the pace and scale of change in organisations may lead purchasers and providers to get distracted from the task of improving services. Much of the guidance and literature on care planning and management is theoretical; there is a lot of exhortation to 'do the right thing' but very little about the practical difficulties faced by both users and professionals. As a result, professionals often find themselves working in isolation, with working days dominated by paperwork rather than helping people's lives improve.

In *Partners in Change*, we share our experience of going beyond the rhetoric, to deliver what users want. We hope that this booklet will:

- help professionals to reflect on their practice and consider new approaches;
- give health and social service commissioners the confidence to question providers about how they deliver services;
- encourage partnerships with service users who often struggle to maintain a precarious existence in the community and deserve better;
- make the voice of direct experience listened to in all parts of the mental health system.

Creating choices

The ideas presented here are drawn from three action-learning programmes established in Clwyd, Leeds and Swindon as part of the King's Fund Better Futures project. These programmes focused on improving quality of life for individual service users, defined in their own terms. Having clear aims enabled us to maintain our focus and prevented us from being knocked off course by the organisational and managerial changes happening all round us. The work covered many of the features of good care programming and care management, including staying in touch, identifying and solving problems, creating choices for people and involving workers in other parts of a service or other agencies.

Although the work in each project area varied in response to local needs and concerns, the three programmes shared the following common aims:

- to enable staff to get to know individual recipients of services as *people* rather than cases;
- to explore in detail their current use of services and existing networks of support;
- to plan ways with the person of improving their quality of life.

All three project areas were in different stages of transition from institutional to community-based services, and each set itself additional goals which included:

- to provide a focus for thinking about the needs of people with serious and long-term difficulties during the transition period;
- to help staff from different agencies and professions understand each other's work and how this links together in a community service;
- to support and learn from each other in carrying out the work;
- to draw out the implications of the work for practice, management and organisation, in order to influence how local mental health services are developed.

In each locality, an action learning group was set up, consisting of professionals from health and social services and the voluntary sector. There were some local variations in membership. In Leeds, two service user consultants joined the group and, in Swindon, a carer consultant took part. The Clwyd group included managers who joined in order to ease the application of lessons learnt from the project work to service development. Each professional participant agreed to work with at least one client, usually someone with whom they were already working, over a twelve-month period.

Why action learning?

There were a number of reasons for establishing action learning groups, including:

- the core values of the project - i.e. the uniqueness of the individual and the need to develop options and choice – could be put into practice through the action learning process;
- professionals from different agencies could enrich their practice and understanding through sharing ideas and information;
- the three projects could provide information about how to develop needs assessment and user-led services. This information would complement existing material on models and content of care management and care programmes.

The action learning process

The action learning groups organised their work along similar lines. Each met regularly over a twelve-month period to review progress and plan the next stage of their work. Between meetings, the members worked with service users on specific tasks and prepared to report back at the next meeting. King's Fund Centre development staff and an independent consultant facilitated these regular meetings.

The basic structure of the work followed this pattern:

- getting the involvement of one or more service users;
- getting to know the person;
- drawing up a personal profile which included strengths and interests as well as needs and wants;
- planning with individual users to achieve what they wanted;
- reviewing action and current and potential service possibilities.

While involved in the work with individual users, the action learning groups also looked at imaginative solutions to meeting need, such as combining service responses with mainstream services open to everyone and working with volunteers and befrienders.

Chapter 2

The policy background

Better Futures was a short-term project, and therefore its action learning programmes were not specifically linked to the local development of the care programme approach (CPA) and care management. The issues raised by CPA and care management, however, provided the background to the Better Futures project as it got under way in 1992. CPA and care management are continuing to evolve and implementation is still not complete in all the localities.

Influences on CPA and care management

The ideas underlying CPA and care management have been around for a long time. Statutory aftercare was first introduced under the Mental Health Act 1983 for people on specific sections, but implementing it, without properly developed community services, always proved difficult. 'Case management' (as 'care management' was previously known) was a feature of the 'Care in the Community' pilot projects funded by the DHSS for people resettled from long-stay institutions. These were evaluated and publicised by the Personal Social Services Research Unit at the University of Kent.[1]

In 1989, Research and Development for Psychiatry (now the Sainsbury Centre for Mental Health) instituted a series of case management projects for people with long-term mental health needs, and evaluation has shown that it can make a positive contribution to people's lives.[2]

Other influences have been the wealth of research literature on case management in mental health coming from the USA, particularly the studies of assertive outreach schemes such as the well-known service in Madison, Wisconsin[3] and its replication in England, at the Maudsley Hospital, London.[4]

Case management was eventually renamed 'care management', not only to reflect the preferences of service users, but also to signal that it has elements of community and service development as well as individual casework.

Care management in the 1990s

Care management was introduced as a local authority duty for all priority service client groups under the NHS and Community Care Act 1990. Implementation was delayed until 1992 to give local authorities more time to prepare. CPA was originally introduced in 1991 for people leaving psychiatric wards and was subsequently extended to cover everyone referred to the specialist psychiatric services. This has led to confusion about who CPA is for and whether everyone needs the same detailed assessment. Links with local authority care management systems have not been particularly clear.

Split services

A care programme includes a social needs assessment if this is relevant, so it would make sense to have a single person responsible for coordinating provision across health and social services. In many places, the staggered start date has allowed health and social services to set up *separate* systems, with the result that an individual may have a keyworker for CPA *and* a care manager. However, where CPA and care management form a single system, it is more common for the NHS to take the leading role, involving social services where necessary. There are similar problems of responsibilities split between agencies in child protection services, and the loose links between health and social services have meant that lessons for mental health services have not been learnt.

Splits in a system which is supposed to deliver coordination and continuity of care undermine CPA in a number of ways. Our work showed the need for both the good relationship and the direct care-giving associated with CPA. It also highlighted the importance of linking with key people in a person's life and with main service areas (e.g. housing), smoothing pathways into leisure and work opportunities and, in some cases, creating new services. The latter activities are more typical of care management. In Wales, interestingly, CPA does not apply because it is felt to be implicit in the role of care coordinator as described in the All-Wales Mental Illness Strategy.

Politics of costs and public concern

The introduction of care management was partly a response to political concern about rising levels of public expenditure as health services transferred the costs of caring for people leaving hospitals to the social security budget. Local authorities must now assess people for community care within limits of a specific social security budget.

Public concern about the perceived dangerousness of people with a severe mental illness also shaped CPA policy. The need for planned follow-up for people leaving psychiatric hospital was first mooted in the Spokes Inquiry (1988) into the killing of social worker Isabel Schwartz. Concern was further heightened by the case of Ben Silcock, the young man who climbed into the lions enclosure at London Zoo and was badly mauled. The Ritchie Inquiry (1994) into the death of Jonathan Zito also highlighted the ease with which people can slip through the net on discharge from hospital. Government response has been to strengthen the protective aspects of CPA through the introduction of a supervised discharge order and supervision registers. One result is that the debate about community care for people in long-term contact with mental health services is being conducted increasingly within a framework of restrictions, rather than improving quality of life and opportunity.

Efficiency and protection of individuals and the community are good objectives as part of a package of aims, but they may amount to fewer options for individuals. More money may go into protection (i.e. keeping people in hospital) than into improving the quality of life of people living in the community. The House of Commons Select Committee (1994) has highlighted inadequate funding of community mental health services in inner cities.

Keeping quality in our sights

The policy initiatives of CPA and care management have therefore had to face a series of difficulties, which has meant professionals coming under increasing pressure in terms of workload and bureaucracy, and managers and commissioners having to adjust to rapid organisational change. In the current climate, risk reduction seems to be a higher priority than making those improvements in someone's quality of life which could sustain them in the longer term. Opportunities offered by new structures of assessment and care planning are therefore being missed.

Action learning addressed these difficulties by turning professional attention to the everyday reality of lives wherein services are being received. Attention to each individual and the fabric of their daily lives meant that new possibilities became visible. Assessments and care planning carried out in action learning environments often generated creative options for service delivery, highlighted unforeseen needs, produced unexpected feedback for commissioners and managers, and pointed to new directions for service development.

Chapter 3

Working with individuals

Each of the action learners undertook to do some detailed work over a twelve-month period with one or more service users, to improve their quality of life. About 20 service users were involved in the three localities, and professionals had contact with another twelve who either withdrew from the programme before it was completed or dropped out because their workers decided to leave.

The service users

In the main, workers invited service users that they already knew to join the programme. All had a history of serious and long-term mental illness and were usually people about whom the workers had some concerns but with whom they had not done any detailed work or had tried and failed. They were living in various sorts of residential care, with parents or in their own accommodation, and most were on long-term medication. Many were not involved with day services.

Explaining the purpose of the action learning programme to service users proved difficult at times. We wanted to make sure that each person understood what was involved and what rights and sanctions they had in controlling the material that was shared in the action learning groups. Inevitably, a lot of time went into explaining a complex and unfamiliar process. The approach that we used in the three localities allowed the work to evolve according to the pace and needs of the individual service user.

Overcoming fear of change

We underestimated how frightening the idea of change could be. For some, even the slightest change could appear to threaten their existing resources such as their homes or benefits. We began to understand how fragile some service users felt that their hold was over their basic life supports and how greatly they worried about losing the little that they had. In general, their everyday experience was one of powerlessness.

For some, the reassurance that improvements in their quality of life could be limited to the very small steps forward that they wanted to make was enough to gain their agreement to participate but, with others, even starting the process of negotiation was impossible. The service users who dropped out of the programmes did so during or at the end of the needs assessment stage, when possibilities of change were being opened up. This suggests the need to carry out this process very slowly over numerous visits and to progress in very small steps at the individual's own pace.

BOX 1
Making contact with Julia

Julia was a client of our team for many years before I was introduced to her. I knew her from conversations with colleagues, and everyone in the team agreed that she seemed suitable for the Better Futures project. I met her first on a joint visit with a community psychiatric nurse (CPN), and we tried to reinforce the fact that I would be working alongside the CPN rather than replacing her. As Julia saw it, she was living a life of dull routine and soon grasped the aims of Better Futures. She was a lively and generous woman, with many interests which she had let lapse over the years.

Initially, I tried to engage her in talking about her enthusiasms, rather than looking at issues which might have appeared closer to her mental illness. This process may have been slow, but the framework of Better Futures enabled me to feel justified in taking time to get to know Julia, and for her to build up confidence in me.

We got to know each other well over the weeks, and the fact that I was not seen as an official, but more as a friend, helped to establish rapport.

Women in long-term services

The majority of the service users invited to join the programme were men (while the majority of the action learners were women). This gender imbalance was unintentional and not recognised until the results of the programme were analysed. This pattern reflects the gender mix in long-term services in some of the Better Futures localities – 70 per cent men and 30 per cent women. This may be due the fact that women develop mental illness later in life and have by then acquired better coping skills. There are other factors too. Women are more likely to seek psychological help, whereas the mainstay of long-term services is help with everyday living. People who have moved into this service area are thought not to benefit from psychological help. There is also evidence from MIND's 'Stress on Women' campaign that women feel uncomfortable in male-designed and dominated services and may choose to stay away.

Much of the literature on working with people with long-term needs stresses the importance of 'engagement' and developing a close relationship. Particular care needs to be taken with women, some of whom will have been abused in the past. In view of current concerns about the potential for abusive relationships between therapist and client, the option for women to have women workers should be made available.

BOX 2
Anne's story

Jo had been Anne's CPN for some time. When she approached her about taking part in Better Futures, Anne initially seemed quite keen. As Jo started to collect information about Anne, she realised that, apart from her symptoms, she knew very little about her. It became clear to Jo, however, that Anne was very distressed by questions about her past and she decided that it was not in Anne's interests to pursue the work. Over the following months, Anne deteriorated and was eventually admitted to hospital. When she came home, she asked Jo if they could take up their work together again. Because of their past experience, Jo felt that she did not have the skills to help Anne and referred her to the psychology service. Pat, a woman psychologist, started seeing Anne every week. She found out that Anne had been sexually abused as a child. The prospect of any close relationship was terrifying to her.

In allowing themselves to be led by service users, professionals had to decide when to step back and when to press ahead. For this reason, professionals using this approach need to be committed to user-centred planning and to have experience of working with people with long-term needs, as well as receiving feedback and support from colleagues, as the action learners did.

Race and culture

Race issues were not really covered in our work. Professionals worked with three individuals from ethnic minority backgrounds. Two of them did not choose to explore their backgrounds, but the third did. Insufficient work was done on this to draw any conclusions, but there is a need, given that black voluntary sector workers were critical of the racial and cultural awareness of white staff, to address this issue more fully.

Getting the whole picture

During the project, the professionals took time to get to know the person with whom they were working, using a variety of methods besides formal assessment. It was difficult for some to accept that they did not already know a person with whom they had been working for a long time but, using different techniques, everyone gathered additional information. We used picture profiles, checklists and life-charts to explore each person's current use of services and existing support networks (see below). We also discussed their present and past experience to find out about their strengths, interests, likes and aspirations (see below). It was not easy for everyone to recognise that by such unconventional means they had achieved a thorough assessment and re-assessment. However, after discussion and support in the action learning group, this way of working was accepted as a valid and professional approach.

Because the assessment is carried out away from formal work settings, care needs to be taken that service users realise that the activity is part of an assessment process and are not caught off guard by the informality of the situation.

BOX 3
Three unconventional assessments

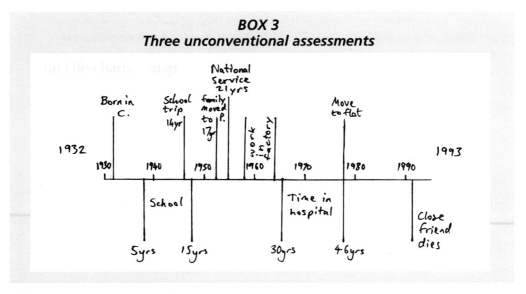

(a) Life-charts map

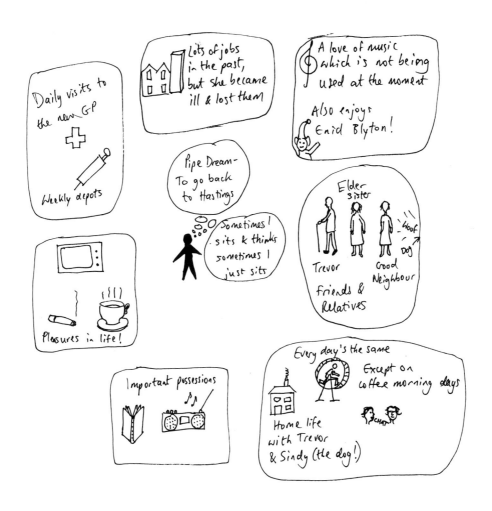

(c)
Jack, a CPN, talks about his work with Clive, a young man living in residential care. At the start of the action learning programme, nothing was happening in his life and he had no desire to do anything.

'I had been working with Clive for some time but, partly because my time was limited and partly because Clive tended to keep his distance, he was not someone I had been able to get close to. He had significant long-term mental health problems, and I was very aware that he was not fulfilling his potential.

Clive had talked with some pleasure about once playing 'pitch and putt' and expressed an interest in doing this again and in learning more about golf. This coincided with one of my own hobbies and seemed to offer an ideal opportunity to meet Clive more informally. There were problems to be overcome concerning cost and equipment, but the enthusiasm was there and a game was set up.

As well as providing Clive with an interesting and rewarding leisure outlet, it offered us the opportunity to develop a relationship which allowed Clive to talk naturally and openly about himself. A picture of his past and of his hopes and needs emerged in the course of normal conversation in a way that would have been unlikely using more structured assessment tools or in a more traditional client–worker relationship. As a result of these encounters, based as they were on a more equal footing, both Clive and I achieved, for the first time, a highly valued relationship and discovered where we were going in our work together'.

As a result of this work, Clive now attends a day centre, takes part in a number of activities in his community and has made some friends. Jack feels that Clive has the potential to develop further.

The need for a variety of assessment tools

Workers found that having a range of tools helped, first of all, in getting the person interested and then in eliciting a fairly comprehensive set of information. For example, pictures could sometimes be more powerful than words in expressing what people wanted to say, and life-charts enabled a person's whole life to be looked at – not just the hospital admissions and periods of living on the edge of society. This part of the work showed that users had a very wide range of needs that were not just health-related (see Fig.1), and therefore any tools used needed to have a holistic focus.

The role of managers

A key factor in the success of this approach was the support and agreement of managers to methods which may be more time-consuming than traditional ones. Permission to test new techniques freed workers to be creative and imaginative. They had the scope to try out alternative assessment methods as part of a range of useful techniques. These could then be used in their everyday work.

Service-related

Place of safety
Rescue from law
Crisis contact point
Psychological assessment & input
Planned and structured support
A psychiatrist who understands
Formal review process recorded,
   agreed, signed
Full assessment (including carer)
Information and update on
   treatment and state-of-the-art
   psychiatry

Support

Someone to listen
Reassurance
Individual attention
Continuous support
Independent advocate
Help in making decisions
   about relationships
Counselling over previous
   relationship
Facilitation of contact with ex-partner
Medication – help to come off
   or stay on
Alternatives to medication

Accommodation

More suitable
Security of tenure
More independent
Privacy

Material

Money
Make-up
Clothes
Regular meals
Cigarettes

Work

Job skills
Career guidance

Day-to-day living

Help with self-care
Financial management
Confidence/assertion
Make own decisions
Small steps towards independence
Coming off medication
Living with or without medication
Self-medication

Close relationships

To be loved/needed
A girlfriend

Socialising and friends

A safe friend
Alcohol-free ordinary social environment
Don't want to always be with people
   like myself

Hobbies/interests

Cats
Watching football
Concessions (not demeaning)
To be able to afford interests

Figure 1 Range of needs identified – Swindon group

Making a plan

The action learning groups used what the individual service user wanted as goals (see Fig.2). Each goal was broken down into often very small steps so that progress was visible, if slow. These steps could be described as problems to be overcome or needs. For example, wanting to move house instantly creates a number of tangible problems which need to be resolved – finding somewhere suitable, buying furniture, budgeting to pay rent and bills, learning to keep house, shop and cook, dealing with repairs. On a more personal level, coping with the stress of moving may be an issue, as well as the need to negotiate new relationships with parents, if the person is moving out of the family home.

Working with what the person wanted did not present major difficulties. People often chose goals that might be difficult to attain quickly but were within the range of ordinary hopes and aspirations. A few were related to the person's mental health problem. Some changes were very small but significant to the individual.

One of the advantages of working towards goals was that it narrowed the range of problems to be solved to those that were immediately relevant. It was easier to track the reason for and content of particular interventions during the year. Without a focus such as this, professional work can be limited to short-term thinking and crisis resolution.

Using a project approach

Breaking the work down into small steps means that professional work can be organised as a series of projects. Peter Huxley has drawn parallels between this way of working and the task-centred social work of the 1970s.[5] There, however, contact with the client terminated with completion of the task; in our model, where the aim is continuity, service user and worker would progress to the next small project.

Pace and style are both crucial in helping users of mental health services meet their objectives. As some workers found, impatience to achieve results is likely to end in failure. Presenting choices and options in a low-key way was more likely to succeed than offering an organised package of care. This suggests that while workers need to be aware of an individual's overall level of need, too much change at one time may feel overwhelming. Working on one goal at a time may be more effective.

Small changes can lead to changes in self-perception

For many years, home for Ted had been a hostel. Though happy living there, he was approached to be part of the Better Futures initiative to help him broaden his options, as life outside the hostel was limited to going to a day hospital. Working with him over the year (life map, identifying interests and goals) revealed many aspects of his life that were not previously known. His goal was modest – he wanted to learn to cook. Managing this fairly quickly, he was then able to enjoy shopping and eating more healthily. Once he could cook, he began to budget for himself, something that had previously caused problems at the hostel.

These seemingly small triumphs, which most of us take for granted, gave him a greater sense of himself. He began to be uncomfortable about going to the day hospital, feeling that it was reinforcing negative ideas about himself.

His goals now include finding things to do outside the hostel and day hospital, following up his interest in gardening and aeroplanes.

Putting the plan into action

For a plan to work, professionals needed to anticipate problems and think of possible solutions. All were working under considerable pressure. Most of the community mental health team workers involved in the programmes had to manage huge caseloads – 50 was quite common. In residential and day care settings, some contended with staffing levels which could not accommodate staff absence or vacant posts.

- Change the way I feel about myself; increase sense of self-esteem
- Learn to be more assertive
- Understand psychiatric diagnosis, its implications and treatment
- Work out what I want out of life
- Budget and cook for myself
- Improve diet
- Find some outside interests
- Manage my finances
- Find an occupation, alternatives to day provision; complete course of study
- Move house

Figure 2 Summary of individual goals – Leeds group

Crisis work with individuals and their families was a way of coping with pressure. It was also 'safer' than working with someone to bring about changes in their life. In a crisis, options are reduced, usually to increasing the person's medication or getting them admitted to hospital. Developing the supports that might keep someone out of hospital brings a whole array of options into play, and it becomes difficult for busy and unsupported professionals to deal with this level of uncertainty. In the new mood of unease about community care, managers may also prefer certainty to risk-taking.

It was not easy for professionals to take the initiative, but it turned out to be essential, particularly where other professionals were involved and there were no formal channels of communication. Professionals called planning meetings to share information and solve problems rather than for routine monitoring purposes.

There is some evidence from the work that service users found this problem-oriented style of meeting easier to attend than care review meetings, even when a large number of people were present. Involving service users in planning meetings and deciding who should be invited help to make multi-professional meetings useful to service users.

Finally, service user consultants in the Leeds action learning group advised that the number of people attending a planning meeting was less of an issue than the venue. It had to be somewhere safe and familiar, but not necessarily the person's home, which might feel too intrusive. The local health centre or a day centre where the person felt comfortable were both possibilities.

Creating choices

Offering service users choices demanded three resources that were in short supply – information, money and time. Most professionals had a working knowledge of statutory services but were sometimes hazy about the voluntary sector.

Information

One of the localities had produced, and one was in the process of producing, a directory of local mental health resources. Not all professionals found such written information particularly helpful in providing options to suggest to service users. They were more likely to refer if they already knew the staff in the other service. This is one of the reasons why information needs to be provided interactively – a person on the end of the telephone as well as a directory, to talk through the options and advise on people to link with.

BOX 5
A planning meeting for Alan

Alan had been offered the tenancy of a flat. Except for some time at college, he had been living with his mother, and things were becoming more difficult at home. Previous attempts to move had failed, and Alan was becoming worried that he would not manage the move this time.

The action learner knew that a number of people were involved with Alan, although they were not in touch with each other. She and Alan called a planning meeting to bring together all the relevant people who could help and support him in the move – his CPN, housing support worker, his GP and his mother. His psychiatrist was also invited to attend but declined.

The meeting was held at the doctor's surgery, a venue that everyone felt comfortable with. All the people present agreed to offer some help or support to Alan in moving house. The tasks identified ranged from buying and moving furniture, decorating and help with budgeting to personal support. His mother turned out to be in favour of the move; until then no one had been sure of her views.

At the meeting, people offered to carry out certain tasks. These were written down and circulated to everyone present. A further meeting was arranged a few weeks later, as support at a time of major change needed to be flexible and responsive. Previously, workers had scaled down contact without realising that there was no input from anyone else. The planning meeting that Alan organised (with help) brought together an effective network which could work at his pace and respond to his strengths and needs.

People come into the mental health services through many different points of entry and often have most contact with staff who lack a formal mental health training. So GPs, housing support workers and day service staff also need access to information and the opportunity to discuss it with someone knowledgeable.

Money

We found that small amounts of money were essential to improve the quality of life of individuals who were existing on welfare benefits. Often, workers would find that they were stuck because they could not find very small sums. People in work tend to take for granted the rising cost of educational and leisure activities and forget that they are beyond the reach of most people on benefits. The following are some of the things that people needed money for:

- gardening tools;
- expenses for trips and outings;
- entrance to a sports centre;
- a computer (or access to one);
- a ticket to a football match;
- some make-up;
- expenses for a volunteer or befriender to accompany two or three people on an outing.

In theory, direct payment was not the only way in which some of these items could have been obtained, but in reality, any alternative method proved difficult and exceedingly time-consuming to organise. For instance, one action learner was working with a user who was a lifelong supporter of his local football club, but he could no longer afford the £15 entrance fee to matches. His worker spent much time trying to extract a concessionary price from the club but to no avail. Another worker put a great deal of effort into contacting charities and training agencies to see if she could get funding for a computer but was also unsuccessful. We concluded that direct access to some funding which could pay expenses for volunteers and befrienders as well as for goods and services was vital to the success of this work.

As a result of Better Futures, Leeds social services has commissioned a pilot flexi-fund to which service users and their keyworkers can apply directly. A panel including service users will decide whether the application meets the criteria for the fund and make the award accordingly. The Leeds scheme is being evaluated to see what contribution it makes to people's quality of life. Other places have devolved budgets to care managers (Nottingham) and to long-term support teams (Lancashire).

Time

The most important resource of all is time. Hard-pressed professionals appreciated the chance which the project offered them to plan their work, but this was very untypical of their normal working life.

Time to support people to do new things and the ability to take a long-term view were crucial in helping some people to bring about change. Having money to do something was not enough on its own. Making the arrangements for people to attend something was also not effective; the service user might attend once or twice (perhaps to please the worker) but would often not continue. Low-key support and a long-term view seem to be the main ingredients in moving forward.

BOX 6
Access to a sports centre

One person's goal was to do more sport. A brainstorming session enabled the action learning group to look at ways in which someone who has great difficulty in being with new people, could make use of the local sports centre.

Barriers to going to the sports centre included an intimidating atmosphere, expense, debilitating side-effects of medication and going somewhere new for the first time. Ideas for overcoming the blocks included encouraging the sports centre to offer low-key, 'safe' sessions at off-peak times, making use of concessions available, developing more flexible sources of funding to pay session fees, finding an 'oppo' – a companion who could share the enthusiasm and be both a support and partner (for badminton or squash). Several ideas about where to find an 'oppo' emerged:

- a council for voluntary service volunteer;
- a volunteer with shared interests;
- a student on a local sports course;
- an 'ad' at the sports centre or by asking at the desk.

Finding the right supporter would involve some detailed and lengthy networking (the action learner did not himself have time to provide this type of support).

Sessional workers, volunteers and befrienders can potentially be used as supporters if some funding is available to support, train and pay expenses. One of the action learning groups considered making use of helpers outside the multi-disciplinary team. Some of the workers had had mostly unhappy experience of volunteers. Volunteers had been misguidedly expected to carry out their tasks without professional input. Projects using volunteers need to invest time in educating ordinary members of the public that are recruited, particularly into allaying their anxieties about media portrayal of mental illness, and professionals need to provide ongoing support for them.

Finally, time might be needed to create new opportunities or services. Most of the things that participants wanted, such as housing and access to mainstream leisure facilities, involved a lot of work to arrange but were quite straightforward. Sometimes people wanted to do something such as gardening where the effort required could not be justified for one person, although it might be possible to develop an allotment for three or four people. Most professionals do not have the time or the skills to set up a scheme of this type. Development officers who might once have done this sort of work are now almost extinct in NHS Trusts; service development is seen as part of the general management role. Development officers are more common in social services but their brief is not always clear. Increasingly, statutory services are looking to the voluntary sector to develop this type of service, but it does depend on professionals being willing to network with voluntary agencies and help them in finding resources.

Interpreting successes and failures

Over the course of the year, a number of people moved house, took up day activities or learned new skills. It would be wrong, however, to credit the action learning programmes alone with these changes since there are so many other influences on people's lives. Nevertheless, the progress made during the year seems to have been positive and service users and workers have made some favourable comments.

The Clwyd programme was evaluated by the Health Services Research Unit at the University College of North Wales.[6] Over the twelve months, individual service users showed an improvement in social functioning. The other two programmes relied on self-evaluation. The return rate of evaluation forms was low from both users and workers. Two were completed by users in Swindon and one in Leeds. The users were appreciative of their workers' efforts on their behalf: 'The worker encouraged me a great deal through the past year, she helped me a lot'. One said that the approach had brought him out of his shell and made life easier.

We learned how important it is to take a long-term view of someone's life when assessing progress and not to be too hasty in interpreting success and failure. For example, a young man was admitted to hospital largely because no alternative accommodation was available. Relationships with his parents were strained, and he had been living a separate life in the family home in very poor conditions. Matters had come to a head when his parents joined a carers' group and realised that their home situation was intolerable. Although it would have been better if the crisis could have been avoided, at least the hospital admission brought the situation to an end and meant that the problems at home had to be sorted out. The admission to hospital might be seen as a turning point leading to a more satisfactory phase of the person's life.

Measures of outcome therefore need to be treated warily. An apparently positive outcome may be achieved with little effort from user or worker. On the other hand, a lot of hard work may result in a seemingly negative outcome, such as an in-patient admission, but this may have a beneficial long-term effect.

Outcomes for action learners

The workers had mixed feelings about the work with individuals. While some of them appreciated the results, they felt that they would not normally have the time to work in this way. One worker commented:

'It made a real difference to a service user and offered reassessment of a long-standing situation. However, we are constrained by time factors (as ever) and for the work to be undertaken thoroughly a great deal of time is needed.'

The action learning programmes challenged the professionals to work in different ways which some found difficult. Barriers to change emerged as:

- denial – 'We're already doing that.'
- distancing – 'These people lack motivation.'
- feeling devalued – 'I am not getting anything out of this.'

It took time for professionals to accept new ideas. Some were not willing to do so and left.

The main benefits identified by workers who participated throughout included:

- more individual-centred work – a focus on the person rather than the forms-driven process of care planning;
- time to anticipate and solve problems, rather than just respond to crises;
- time to produce creative options;
- the opportunity to practise new techniques – in particular, people's life stories were used to good effect.

Outcomes for user consultant action learners

The user consultants in the Leeds action learning group learned that professionals do not have all the answers. In their interactions with professionals, users can often receive the impression that they do. In reality, professionals and users need to work together to find answers, with service users feeling empowered to bring their own ideas about solutions to meetings with professionals.

Individual care planning – tricks and traps for practitioners

Assessment

- Take time to get to know the person.
- Try different ways of eliciting and recording information.
- Try different settings away from your base.
- Find out about the person's strengths and interests as well as their needs and problems. For example, have they had a job in the past? If so, what skills did they use? Have they had any hobbies or interests? What do they enjoy doing at the moment?
- Resist the temptation to make assumptions about what the person is capable of.
- Remember that any change can appear threatening, particularly if past experiences of change have not been good.

Planning

- Find out what the person wants and agree a way forward.
- Break the work down into many small steps.
- Allow time for the person to take in new ideas and get used to them.
- Do not jump in and make all the arrangements yourself; allow the person to go at their own pace.
- Allow them to rethink and change their mind about what they want to do.

Resources

- Try to find some funding for activities and equipment.
- Do offer support, or find someone else to do so, when change is happening; giving someone the resources without the time to support them seldom works.
- Involve other workers where appropriate; be realistic about your own skills and do not try to meet all the person's needs yourself.

Organising the work

- Plan, plan, plan! Anticipate and solve problems; do not wait for crises to happen.
- Work on one goal at a time.
- Organise the work into small projects so that you know why you are visiting the person and what you are working on together.

Linking with other people

- Get to know the people who run the services that you want to use.
- Involve the person with whom you are working in communications with other people.
- Face-to-face communication is often more powerful than a telephone call or letter.
- Call planning meetings to provide extra support when needed and solve current problems rather than wait for the routine care review meeting.

Chapter 4

Issues for professionals

Attitudes and techniques

The essence of this kind of mental health work is the ability to see service users as people, and this often means a shift in workers' attitudes. Many workers took time to accept that they did not know people with whom they had been working, sometimes, for a very long time. They found that they needed to learn new techniques, including:

- using empowering methods of assessment;
- planning the work around goals and objectives;
- being proactive in solving problems and, when necessary, contacting key people (with the person's permission);
- learning how to use information about local resources;
- making links with other workers and services;
- developing new services.

These techniques are administrative and developmental and, on the surface, might seem to be outside the range of what is normally considered to be the professional skills required for work of this kind. Yet in reality, this type of work is highly skilled, drawing on reserves of judgement and experience. Risk assessment sits somewhere between the skills listed above and the following:

- up-to-date knowledge of medication – its purpose, effects and side-effects;
- ability to give advice on reduced and intermittent use of medication;
- crisis planning; many service users now like to use crisis cards, and key-workers need to keep a record of what the user wants;
- psychological and self-help approaches to managing communications within families, sharing information and coping with 'voices';
- knowledge of welfare benefits.

Not all professionals need to be expert in every skill, but each team of workers needs to have a clear idea of the competences required to work with people with long-term needs and to either develop those competences within the team or know where to access them.

Action and vulnerability

In one group in particular, the issue of staff vulnerability quickly came to the fore. Some professionals were anxious about revealing the detail of their work to other people. They were used to a 'policeman's notebook' style of reporting within their staff groups and found it difficult to share their work in depth with workers from a wide spectrum of agencies.

Sometimes underlying such anxieties lay uncertainty about the limits of the professional role. There were instances of workers going along with stuck family situations ('I think his family copes with him very well'), which would then lead to the inevitable crisis. Some episodes also showed that not all workers were good at assessing risk. In general, they were practised at knowing when someone required intensive support. Some were less good at seeing the long-term risk inherent in certain situations involving families or neighbours, or risks to physical health. Again, a lot could be learned from child protection services about assessing risk in a fragmented system. This stresses the need for coordination of professional input and clear, open channels of communication.

This does not mean that professionals should interfere without being asked in all aspects of a person's life. It might be appropriate to give constant feedback on the reality of the situation to the person or family and to make low-key, unpressurising suggestions about ways of resolving a difficult situation.

Sharing with colleagues was often encouraging and allowed workers to take more risks. For example, in a planning meeting with a service user and other workers, a CPN was able to ask the service user if her mother could contact him if she became aware of any problems. The CPN had very infrequent contact with the service user when she was well and had no way of knowing when extra support was needed.

Setting goals

The locality groups used what individuals wanted as the goals which they worked towards. This may raise objections, including:

- users do not know what they want;
- users want things that are unrealistic;
- users change their minds about what they want.

Many people, put on the spot, would be hard put to say what they want. Part of an empowering assessment process would be to help people to explore what they want, perhaps by trying out a number of opportunities and services to find out what suits them best. This is a dynamic, continuing process, which might last for a year or more. The need for a lengthy assessment period should not preclude all change in the meantime (for example, making someone stay in hospital until the process is completed). On the contrary, it can provide the background of continuity necessary for someone to identify important changes they want in their life and begin to make them.

Very few people wanted things that were completely unrealistic. On the whole, they had low expectations and tended to be unambitious. Sometimes, goals could be aimed for but would not be achieved for many years if at all. For example, one participant's wish to 'get married' might seem a long way off but his need to gain confidence in mixing with other young people and to make friends of both sexes could be reasonably accommodated. These were necessary steps to achieving what he wanted.

Some people did need to stop and reconsider their goals, perhaps because of a change in their situation. Owing to the continuing assessment process, most people had the opportunity to become clearer about what they wanted and generally stuck to this during the year.

Networking and the development role

' Do you want to know what has really improved my quality of life? ...
Disabled Living Allowance. '

For most mental health professionals, the traditional model of work with service users is one-to-one, the out-patient interview, the flying home visit. People's needs cannot be easily encompassed within this model. A skilled and sympathetic worker, able to access other agencies and resources when necessary, can make a lot of difference to people's lives.

Professionals often felt that they had to try to meet all of a user's needs themselves even when they did not have all the skills to do so. Knowing when to call on the skills of other professionals or seek expert advice from welfare or housing specialists is an important skill in its own right. Professionals were unsure about the boundaries of their role and were sometimes reluctant to take the initiative in communicating and liaising with other workers, particularly outside their own agency.

In order to offer people choices, professionals need to know what is available locally in statutory, voluntary and mainstream services. For example, the church hall group addressing the welfare needs of the local black community may be more appropriate and acceptable to a black user than a standard mental health day centre. Without good information networks, such informal, self-help community groups are sometimes more difficult to identify but they may appropriately meet a user's needs.

Helping someone to access services is part of offering choice, but sometimes the service or opportunity that is required does not exist. One way of developing new options is for two or three professionals to work together on a project such as an allotment, which three or four service users could work on, or a weekend support scheme.

The Clwyd Better Futures group used their King's Fund Centre grant to fund small service developments worked up by community mental health teams. Small sums of money – up to £5000 over two years, but often much smaller sums – were available to support these developments. The most successful projects involved users, carers and the voluntary sector. The Clwyd teams also took the opportunity to develop direct links with local colleges, training agencies and employers. (They found that they could not rely on intermediary agencies, such as the Department of Employment, to make the connections for them.) Working with colleagues in this way can help to foster a team's cohesiveness and sense of purpose.

Chapter 5

Management perspectives

Partners in Change has implications for managers and this chapter is particularly addressed to middle managers.

Just as professionals need to work proactively with their clients, managers also need to be proactive in managing the service. When individual professionals have been working in a service for a long time and acquired a fair amount of autonomy, it is sometimes difficult to manage assertively. Team-building strategies, such as the learning forum described below and team projects where members cooperate on tasks, may help. Multi-agency training, involving service users and the voluntary sector may also have a part to play.

Making time

The approaches described here require time. We found that some managers were unsympathetic to complaints of work overload and, in order to cope, professionals managed their workloads defensively. They gave some service users low priority and saw them infrequently so as to make time for people who were of immediate concern. They did not discharge people (which would have made the prioritisation explicit) since this would lead to managers adding a new case, needing more active work, to their workload.

Within residential or day care services, there is often conflict between time spent working with an individual and managing the day-to-day fabric of the service. Staffing levels are not adequate or flexible enough to accommodate for vacant posts and absences. Work often proceeds at the pace of the service rather than that of the service user.

Many people who would benefit from long-term specialist mental health services in the community are stuck in the areas of acute provision, where the approaches described here are hard to maintain.

Reducing the workload

Experiences in Better Future localities (and also national indications) suggest that two types of management response would be appropriate to this central resource issue. First, workloads need to be reduced. Individual workloads of between 8 and 20 people in specialist mental health teams would allow for the intensive assessment, planning and development of networks and resources which we recommend. Local negotiation of workload size will depend on complexity of needs, vulnerability of service users and the existence of complementary resources and support networks.

Identifying priorities

Second, the people who would benefit from this kind of assessment and care planning should be identified and prioritised. Workers in all settings offering services to people with on-going and serious mental health problems, would have a small number – two or three – of designated people who were judged as likely to benefit from this approach, to work with. People who will potentially be subject to new restrictive mental health legislation seem to be particularly appropriate for this way of working.

Decisions about priorities need to be made openly. If someone has good support and is managing well, there may be no need for secondary mental health service involvement. Explicit negotiations between service user and worker can produce agreements about reviewing progress and also about who may contact the service if the person needs extra support. Many service users like to do this through a crisis card on which the worker can keep a record. If contact is cut back and no markers are set to alert a team that a user may need more support for a time, their next contact with the person is likely to be as an in-patient.

Managers with a realistic view of the timescales required to work positively with people are crucial to the development of services for people with continuing needs. Many of the professionals who took part in the action learning programmes felt that managers were more often interested in throughput than in achieving quality outcomes for individuals. Managers are also under pressure but do need to listen and learn from the experiences of workers. They also need to collect evidence about the outcomes of different patterns of work in order to justify any changes in activity levels to senior managers and purchasers.

Sometimes it is possible to create time for detailed work with a small number of individuals by making use of groupwork and consultation skills. Running a group with a colleague from outside the secondary mental health service is an opportunity to share skills and increase the competence of non-specialist workers. Consulting with primary care workers about people with whom they are having difficulties may be a more appropriate response and use of time than accepting a referral to the secondary service.

Encouraging a team or group of workers to share the task of making links with the services that users might want to access is a cost-effective approach. If this task is shared, it need not be time-consuming and will pay dividends in improved communication and cross-fertilisation of ideas, as well as more choice for service users.

Personal development and learning

The successful implementation of individual care planning often requires a cultural change within services; the support of managers is essential to bring this about.

The action learning group provided a model of how opportunities could be provided for professionals to learn from their work, help each other to plan ahead and anticipate problems. Although some professionals found it difficult to share the detailed content of their work, there was evidence that working with others was a generally supportive experience, which enabled professionals to be more adventurous.

As a rule, team clinical meetings are too cursory to allow much real sharing to take place. Without overloading workers with meetings, some better ways need to be found to provide mutual help and shared learning. A forum meeting every two or three weeks might fill the learning gap without taking too much time.

Managers should develop a clear view of the range of competences required to provide a service to people with long-term needs and should devise a training strategy to meet them. Without a strategy, workers going on an ad-hoc collection of training courses may be a costly way of achieving little.

Supervision

Good supervision is essential if professionals are to develop in their role and feel supported in their work. The underlying purpose of supervision is to ensure that a worker is competent and able to do their job. In supervision, the manager seeks to maximise both competence and efficiency by:

- developing personal competence either through allowing the worker to reflect on and learn from their work or by identifying gaps in knowledge and experience which can be met through training;
- helping to manage individual workloads by making explicit decisions about prioritisation and discharge;
- helping to assess risk;
- providing support and a sounding board for ideas.

Multi-agency training

Sharing ideas and learning across agency boundaries can be a powerful way of increasing creativity and confidence. There are two ways of creating multi-agency learning opportunities – through conventional training courses and events and through shared projects.

Joint training

Joint training between health and social services is now becoming more common. Multi-agency training, involving both users and the voluntary sector, is not yet on the agenda. The case for wider involvement in training is that many people from a wide range of agencies and service users themselves have a part to play in providing a coordinated service to people with long-term needs. They need to share their understanding and experiences and develop common working methods and protocols. We found that people such as residential care workers and general practitioners, who had the least training in working with people with long-term needs, often had the most contact with service users. Because there is so little investment in developing such networks, a great deal of potential remains locked away.

Shared projects

Shared projects are another way of crossing agency boundaries. Projects can be quite small – organising a meeting or running a working group – or produce service developments. The advantage of a project approach is that the task has to be clarified and the amount of time required can be defined in advance.

Managing the work with individuals

Work with individuals must be based on a care plan with clear goals. A work pattern of 'maintenance' visits with periodic bursts of crisis intervention is likely to be unsatisfactory for both worker and user. Organising the work around goals or outcomes means that is possible to measure progress, however small, and ask relevant questions about setbacks and problems.

Information and money are vital resources in enabling professionals to work with service users on improving their quality of life. Written information about resources and services in the statutory and voluntary sector has limitations since professionals may be reluctant to refer to someone that they do not know. Some easily accessible money needs to be part of the care plan. A small budget held at team level will pay for activities and equipment and possibly expenses for volunteer befrienders. A larger budget can be used to employ sessional workers to meet more individualised needs, such as a worker who speaks the same language or providing support to a parent in keeping their child at home.

Planning for flexibility and continuity

Many of the people with whom we worked do not fit easily into the standard nine-to-five community mental health team model. They were often reluctant to use day services and a few led unconventional lives, moving from place to place but always coming back. Some only needed to be in touch with secondary services at times of crisis.

It is a great challenge to provide a service to people whose needs are not routine. Managers need to ensure that their systems are able to cope with irregular participation. In one locality, we found that people who 'disappeared' for a time were discharged. When they returned, they had to be re-referred before they could get specialist help and in the meantime, the accident and emergency department was their only source of help. In another locality, the CPNs routinely discharged people who were admitted to hospital, thus making the whole process of discharge planning and identifying a keyworker difficult. Services organised like this seem designed to make service users look like 'difficult customers', when it is the service itself which needs sorting out.

Chapter 6

Commissioning change

Commissioners of services have a crucial role to play in the delivery and development of high-quality, comprehensive and integrated services. This section links our work on individual care planning to more strategic concerns.

Assessment and care planning are fundamental to identifying appropriate service responses for people with serious and continuing needs, and should not be separated from the rest of the service. The emphasis on forms, reviews and computerised statistics makes it seem as though they can. The first requisite for successful care planning is that the elements of a comprehensive service are in place but, by itself, this is not enough. Good systems also need to be in place which allow people both inside and outside the mental health service to communicate, liaise and work cooperatively together.

Changing service content and systems will inevitably have an impact on the staffing, management and culture of mental health services. This may seem like a daunting agenda for the very small number of people involved in commissioning mental health services. What can commissioners achieve?

Strategy and planning

Health and local authorities have key roles in creating a shared vision of how local mental health services should evolve. From this long-term vision an integrated strategy for the development of, and change to, community-based services can be created. The services commissioned should reflect the strategic direction. It is crucial that commissioners take account of the concerns and interests of service users, their families and friends in every aspect of their work. Successful individual care planning for people with ongoing needs involves:

- provision of continuums of health and social care;
- access to a range of ordinary community facilities;
- the development and support of people's ordinary networks.

Joint mental health strategies and the development of jointly commissioned services can ensure that these elements are available. The most important function of a strategic document is to describe the direction that local services should take, rather than how the strategy should be implemented. This is not always well understood, witness the manager who was called away from a Better Futures meeting to attend an 'emergency' strategy meeting.

The strategy is a working tool which can change as circumstances and knowledge alter and it should not act as a barrier to opportunistic development.

Commissioners need to purchase an integrated continuum of care ranging from protective environments to care at home. At the present time, most resources are still tied up in hospitals, although the majority of people with long-term needs live in the community.

Commissioning and service development

The role of commissioners and their relationships with providers are still evolving. We would like to see commissioners take an active role in service development, working alongside providers to change services. The channels for change that are currently open to commissioners – needs assessment for populations, contracting and competitive tendering – are not enough to bring about the changes in culture and practice that we advocate. Change needs to start with developmental relationships, and commissioners can begin to develop these by working closely with others on major service changes, such as individual care planning. From this cooperation can come a detailed understanding of what is needed. This can then be reflected in service specifications and contracts. A contract can reflect particular concerns of service users and specify 'items', such as the option for women to have women therapists and for women-only space to be provided in hospitals and residences. 'Spot' contracting, usually done by social services commissioners, can provide very individualised care packages for people and small-scale, localised responses to identified need.

Deciding on priorities

Responsibilities for commissioners include deciding which client group(s) to prioritise. The number of central directives that have to be implemented makes it imperative that services for people with serious and long-term mental health problems are a high priority.

In thinking about numbers of people requiring a service, commissioners will want to look at morbidity rates (the expected number of people with mental health problems) and compare this with the actual number using services. There is always a difference between morbidity rates and actual use of services but, if there is a large gap or over-representation of particular groups in parts of the service, some further investigation is needed. The Better Futures work highlighted the fact that the majority of people with long-term needs do not use specialised services such as day hospitals/centres or specialist community teams. A rough calculation in one of the localities showed that about 10 per cent of people with continuing care needs were being cared for by specialist community teams and services. Another 10 per cent were in hospital. It must be assumed that the remaining 80 per cent were being served by acute community mental health teams, primary care staff and the voluntary sector, or were not receiving a service at all. Calculations were based on the formula of two people with severe mental health problems per 1000 suggested by the Mental Health Task Force.[7]

The number of people on care programmes may not be a reliable guide as not everyone who requires coordinated care has a care programme.

Individual care planning

Individual care planning should guide the purchasing process. It is crucial that commissioners' perspective and level of planning are linked to the planning work with individuals.

Because most of this work is carried out within a one-to-one relationship, it is not easy for commissioners to understand what is happening. It is however possible to make some assumptions on the basis of activity levels, working methods and staff skills. Action learning groups made this process visible, and issues highlighted by the individual care planning work were taken up locally to produce specific, responsive developments.

The action learning groups highlighted areas in which commissioners need to ask tough questions of providers, especially about workload, timescales, inclusive services, management and styles of working.

Workload

Workload is dictated not only by the number of cases per professional, but also by the needs of service users and the intensity of the work. Depending on the vulnerability of users, and the context of work, workloads of 8–20 people are realistic to enable positive work to be done. Large caseloads lead to 'hidden' prioritisation with resources going to those in crisis.

Timescales

Timescales for achieving results also need to be realistic. Although filling in an assessment form may take an afternoon, helping someone to understand what they want out of life and make real choices could take a year or more. This does not mean that an individual's immediate needs (such as for housing) should be put on hold while they explore long-term life goals. Commissioners need to understand that assessment and review are a continuing process and there is no substitute for time spent with the person. They also need to understand that services for people with long-term needs cannot be time-limited and throughput is not a good measure of productivity.

Responsive services

Commissioners should check that services are inclusive and that women or people from black and minority ethnic groups are not deterred from using them.

Working on an outreach basis means that people can be helped in a more individual way, at least initially. Services that are centre-based are not very effective at reaching vulnerable people. Working with people at home or in places they normally go to may be more helpful.

Organisational issues

Throughout the Better Futures work a range of resources were identified as important contributions to flexible and responsive services. These include the following.

- A variety of professionals to work with people who may have complex needs. As well as professionals, teams which include generic workers can provide more of the practical support that people need over a longer period, including evenings and weekends. The aim should be a 24-hour on-call service, although this may be difficult to achieve initially.
- A fund which can be easily accessed by users and workers, held either at team level or centrally. The fund would increase the range of choices for service users and could be used to pay for activities and equipment as well as expenses for volunteer befrienders.
- Strategies for team and individual workload management able to make time for detailed individual work.
- Clear referral and discharge criteria and explicit prioritisation systems which do not place individuals at risk.
- Services with an understanding of the attitudes and competences required to work with people with long-term needs, and a strategy for bridging the gaps, through training or other means.

Commissioners need to have some knowledge of interventions that have been shown to be effective and that service users feel are helpful. Building up a network of contacts to increase the inevitably limited experience of individual commissioners is a good strategy for meeting gaps in knowledge and developing their confidence about purchasing decisions.

The key areas where people can become lost to the system are the relationships between parts of a service or between agencies. The most crucial interfaces are between hospital and community and between health and social services. Understanding how these work locally is very important. Proactive commissioning can create bridges between services, since it is usually the organisational system that is at fault, rather than the service user. Multi-agency groups in the project areas, including users and carers, used information from local action learning groups to respond to the problem areas identified. They looked at areas such as the relationships between local primary health care and community mental health teams, and between hospital and community services.

In both hospital and community settings, there is often quite intensive work going on but poor mechanisms to keep each other informed and pass on information. For example, in one locality, a professional working closely with a service user and his family in the community, was surprised to meet him as an in-patient in the hospital.

This is an area where detailed questions need to be asked and detailed answers given. In response to a question about discharge planning, an answer such as 'Our CPNs are always on the wards' or 'A social worker attends all ward rounds' is not very clear. A more helpful answer would be: 'Our policy is that the keyworker will carry out an initial assessment within 48 hours of admission and convene the first discharge planning within seven days.' Other important interfaces that the Better Futures work stressed, and about which commissioners should be asking questions, are relationships with:

- users individually and collectively;
- relatives, carers and friends;
- other community teams (e.g. acute, rehabilitation);
- primary care;
- the voluntary sector;
- community groups (including black and ethnic minority groups and women's groups).

The final organisational issue for commissioners is referral and discharge policies. Referral criteria, particularly to specialist teams, should not select out people with the most severe problems. Discharges need to take place because someone no longer needs a service, not because they are currently using a different part of the service or their lifestyle does not fit in with service organisation.

Monitoring and evaluation

Good coordinated information systems are vital tools, particularly for identifying potential long-term need as well as the impact of hospital closure and the changes in service provision on the lives of people currently using services. Collecting the data opposite will help establish in what way people use services.

Some of this information is already collected routinely. Commissioners may wish to collect other elements for specific planning projects. Providers need this information in order to offer a service and commissioners may wish to make sure that they are collecting it or have a plan to do so.

Outcomes

Professionally defined outcomes

Evaluation is essential if we are to provide meaningful care programmes which really are flexible and responsive to need. Clinical audit provides an opportunity for professionals and users to investigate the effectiveness of care in relation to a wide range of factors, and to develop working methods in response to information generated through the audit cycle.

It is important to be specific about the aims of our work, and clinical audit can help to clarify how these aims can be realised. Services will have many different aims for the client group as a whole, and service users will have goals which are specific to them as individuals. Both can be evaluated through the use of clinical audit. (See Fig.3.)

User-defined outcomes

Partners in Change describes elements of user-led care planning. The outcome of the work was defined by the individual service users themselves, in the context of their strengths, aspirations and potential. Monitoring progress towards each personal goal meant that professional intervention could be negotiated, appropriate and responsive to the current situation.

If interventions are based solely on professional perceptions of problems, professional responses and outcomes are produced. A comment from a service user in one of the localities illustrates this:

'According to you as workers, I'm a success because I have a place of my own, am a member of MIND and take part in social activities. In fact, I'm hanging on by my fingernails and I can't easily get the daily help I need to keep going. Every day is a struggle.'

Data set

In-patient information

Referral and discharge policies
Number of admissions
Average length of stay
Use of Mental Health Act
Maximum and minimum length of stay
Number of stays longer than 3 months
Number of repeat admissions by person over 12-month period

Out-patient information

Number of attendances
Average number per session
Number of non-attendances (1st appointment)
Number of non-attendances (2nd appointment)

Same information for day services.

Community services information

Number of people on CPA, s.117 of the Mental Health Act 1983
and supervision registers
Comparison of names on CPN and social services workload with previous
in-patients
Analysis of discharge plans

Primary care

Number of people with long-term needs registered with GPs
Comparison with people on CPN and social services workload

An example of an audit mechanism for evaluating work
with one service user may relate to quality of life:

eg. Maxine aims to increase her leisure activities

STRUCTURE	PROCESS	OUTCOME	AUDIT METHOD
Clear assessment of Maxine's leisure needs	Carry out assessment with Maxine Identify Maxine's perception of her needs Formulate goals eg. to spend one day a week away from the hostel eg... eg...	Implement goal plan eg. swimming on Tuesday with Kate (keyworker) eg... eg... eg...	Record when Maxine goes swimming Record reasons why Maxine doesn't go swimming (eg. pool closed not enough staff family visit) Administer Lancashire QoL Profile (leisure Domain) Repeat and review every 3 months

Fig.3

Conclusion

The action learning projects highlight the importance of ongoing and interactional assessments in the planning of community care for individuals. Such assessments reveal the complex needs and wishes of people with long-term and serious mental health problems, and raise questions as to the quality of services that they receive. The issue of time, of pressures of work, of the importance of defending spaces in which service users and professionals can communicate more fully, recurs constantly and suggests a specific course of action for all professionals concerned to deliver quality services.

Also important were the feedback and support that workers received from colleagues, which gave professionals the confidence to use their initiative, support individuals in making changes in their lives and come up with creative solutions to problems. The evidence is that such work has a wide range of benefits, for individuals, professionals and service delivery systems. It forges networks, encourages different ways of working, develops partnerships and creates positive and unexpected change.

Where commissioners plan for such work, and managers support its continuation, professionals can help improve the quality of people's lives and their own work by making visible what formerly could not be seen.

Appendix 1

Protocol for approaching service users

Each member of the action learning set is requested to make contact with one-to-three individuals with serious and long-term mental health problems at the start of the programme. The aim is to try out a different style of working in which the professional gets to know the individual as a whole person, attempts to understand their needs and wants from their point of view and works out with them a plan for meeting those needs. In the second part of the set, we will look at resources used and organisational barriers to meeting individual needs, but it is really during the first part of the set and subsequent dissemination of the lessons learnt where confidentiality is an issue. The people contacted will need to know:

The purpose of the action learning programme

- to improve the quality of life of a small number of people with serious and long-term mental health problems;
- to learn more about achieving continuity of care for individuals by sharing experiences with other professionals and service users.

The content of the work

- you will spend some time with each individual at home or in the service settings that they use regularly in order to get to know them;
- you will think together about what the person needs in order to improve their quality of life and ways of achieving it;
- you will do some thinking with professionals from other disciplines and agencies during meetings of the action learning set about the person's needs and how best to meet them;
- you and the individual may need to involve other people (professionals and others) in order to achieve the goals that you have identified together.

What we mean by confidentiality

- names and other identifying details will not be revealed outside the action learning group;

- trust is an important part of confidentiality; we will not step outside the person's wishes;
- we will respect the person's privacy and only reveal information about them and their situation after discussing it with them first;
- the person will know what is said about them;
- only relevant information about individuals will be given in the action learning group;
- in certain very exceptional circumstances, other duties and responsibilities may override the duty of confidentiality;
- the same points apply to other professionals that we may come across in the course of the action learning work.

Arrangements for preserving confidentiality within the action learning programme

- only information that has been discussed with the individual will be revealed;
- details that they do not wish revealed will remain private;
- they will be spoken of respectfully at all times.

Arrangements for preserving confidentiality outside the action learning programme

- participants may use stories about individuals to illustrate lessons from the programme, but every care will be taken to conceal the identity of individuals;
- care will be taken to ensure that lessons about the work are disseminated in a way which does not invade the privacy or personal lives of the individuals involved.

Working through the protocol

All of the above will have to be discussed at some length and you may need to make several visits or have several contacts before the person can understand what is involved and agree that they want to be part of it. You may wish to work through the contents of the protocol in a different order from the way in which they are laid out above. Communicating a complex piece of information like this is a very high-level skill and you should use your judgement about how much the person can take in at one time and whether to persist with getting their agreement if their initial reaction is negative. The important thing at this stage is to develop a trusting relationship so that the work you do together has a chance of being effective.

Appendix 2

Areas of people's lives checklist

Background

What is the person's history?
What are the key points in their life?
In what ways and how successfully has the person been involved with mental health services in the past?
How have their culture and race affected their lives and their experience of receiving mental health services?

Relationships

What are the relationships in their life?
Are they involved with family or relatives?
Who are the people who care for them (service providers but also friends, neighbours, shopkeepers – anyone who has shown care and support)?

Personal status

What is the person's view of their own worth?
Do they feel valued by other people?
What choices and decisions, both large and small, can they make about their lives?

Home environment

How much personal space does the person have?
Is it easy to get around on public transport from where they live?
Is their home warm and comfortably furnished?
Do they have sufficient household equipment (e.g. for cooking, laundry)?
Do they have any personal possessions (e.g. photos, gifts)?
Do they have a pet?

Places and activities

Over a week, how does the person spend their time? (Look at evenings and weekends as well as 9–5 activities)
Where do they spend their time?

Preferences

What does the person like doing and find motivating?
What activities do they have negative feelings about?

A desirable future

What do they want out of the future, e.g. more activities, a job, friends, somewhere better to live?
What will happen if nothing changes?
What will help the person to get what they want?
What will get in the way?

Some suggestions for using the checklist

- Treat the document as a guide rather than a questionnaire.
- Try to memorise the sections or use it for reference.
- Use the document in the order that seems appropriate rather that working through each section in turn.
- Try to find out what the person (and their family) want; try not to make too many early assumptions about this.
- Focus on the person's strengths, ambitions and interests; these are the assets that you can build on.
- Treat this assessment as a new beginning; you will probably have already carried out a needs assessment with the person and be only too aware of their problems. Be objective about this process.
- If the person finds it difficult to express themselves, spend some time with them (with their agreement) in different settings to get some of the information that you need.
- Reflect on the process as you go along. Think about whether it feels different and what you liked and disliked about it.

References

1. Challis D, Davies B. Case management in community care. An evaluated experience in the home care of the elderly. Personal Social Services Research Unit. London: Gower, 1986.

2. Ford R *et al*. Implementing case management: Research report on the process of developing case management services for people with a long-term mental illness. London: RDP, 1993.

3. Stein L, Test MA. Alternatives to mental hospital treatment I. Conceptual model treatment program and clinical evaluations. Archives of General Psychiatry 1980; 37:392–7.

4. Myers-Davies S, Wood H. Making community care a user-centred service. Openmind 1994; 67, Feb–Mar.

5. Huxley P. Social work practice in mental health. Aldershot: Gower. 1988.

6. Crosby C. Evaluation of the King's Fund Better Futures action-learning initiative in Clwyd. Health Services Research Unit. University College of North Wales, 1993.

7. Mental Health Task Force. Local systems of support: A framework for purchasing for people with severe mental health problems. London: Department of Health, 1994.

Skill Typewriting

Alfreda M Patten, FSBT

Keyboard Training

Pitman

Skill Typewriting

Keyboarding

PITMAN PUBLISHING
128 Long Acre, London WC2E 9AN

A Division of Longman Group UK Limited

© Alfreda M. Patten 1970, 1978

Fourth edition 1978
Reprinted 1980, 1982, 1983, 1984, 1986, 1987, 1988, 1992

Printed and bound in Singapore

ISBN 0 273 01194 4

Preface

This fourth edition of Skill Typewriting has been completely re-designed. Envelopes, letters, manuscript work and the RSA examination papers have been omitted in order to allow for a more detailed study of the mastery of the keyboard.

Elite paragraphs have been omitted and replaced by new ones in pica type, thus giving a larger variety of practice material - in fact, almost double the quantity of the previous edition.

The material on numbers and upper-case characters has been brought up to date, and additional, timed and more difficult practice given later in the book.

The copying passages on Pages 34-39 inclusive, range from 24 to 105 wpm.

A new feature of Skill is the addition of a set of drills designed to help students to eradicate common errors. These drills are timed, and graded in difficulty and length.

When adding new copying material much thought has been given to the content, in order to expand the students' knowledge of the use of the typewriter, including the lesser employed levers, i.e. the page-line indicator, the half-space, space bar, and the half-space liner. The method of correcting errors by the replacement of words which are one letter shorter (or longer) than the original words is explained, and proportional spacing has a mention. There is a different and clearer arrangement for Roman numerals, and the typing of superior and inferior characters is set out in detail.

Finally, in place of the RSA examination papers there is copying material in varying lengths.

Teachers' Supplement

(See Pages 25(a) to (f).)

Horse brasses, which are now just collectors' items, were,   **12**
in ancient times, badges of ownership, as well as being   **22**
symbols of superstition, or good luck, or protection from   **33**
the 'evil eye', sickness, calamity or death. An unadorned   **45**
disc was a relic of sun worship. Amulets, too, were worn   **56**
for the same reasons. The Romans decorated their belts   **67**
with them and one of the first found here is in a museum   **78**
in Hull.   **80**
The designs on the brasses were of animals and birds, (such   **92**
as the dog, phoenix, eagle, griffin and elephant), the signs   **104**
in the heavens, (sun, moon and stars), regimental crests,   **115**
Prince of Wales' feathers, or tudor rose. The tavern signs   **127**
were also depicted, ie a castle, crossed keys, a crown, a   **138**
beehive, an anchor, tuns or barrels, a crescent, a horse-   **149**
shoe, hearts, a hand clasping a hammer, sheaves of corn,   **160**
and so on.   **162**
The Latten bells (latten meaning brass or bronze), were   **173**
worn by horses, so that the sound of them would warn   **184**
oncoming traffic in the narrow winding lanes.   **194**
Two men owned a foundry in Birmingham as early as 1715 and   **206**
the brasses they produced were sold at fairs by travelling   **218**
salesmen. Commemorative badges were also struck for   **229**
royalty and other famous people.   **236**
If you wish to collect these interesting brasses, you   **247**
must distinguish between those made before 1850, which   **258**
were in heavy metal and weighed approximately four ounces,   **270**
and were carefully produced and well finished, and the   **281**
mass-produced modern ones which are, of course, of little   **292**
value and are not made with the craftsman's expertise.   **303**

Contents

A stenotyping machine is small, portable, silent in	10
operation and is suitable for recording lectures and the	21
business of conferences and meetings.	29
The machine can be placed on the lap when in use, and the	41
operator taps several keys with both hands simultaneously,	53
each set of sounds representing the phonetic syllable of	64
a word. The first letter of the syllable is struck with	75
a finger of the left hand on the left side of the	85
keyboard, the vowels, arranged in the centre front, are	96
manipulated by the thumbs, and the final consonant is	107
struck by a finger of the right hand, on the right side	118
of the keyboard. The three sounds of each syllable are	129
typed with one movement on to the paper roll, which is	140
only about four inches wide. The left-hand consonant	151
appears on the left edge of the paper, the vowels in the	162
middle and the final consonant at the right edge. As the	174
syllable is typed, the paper moves up automatically for	185
the next line - there is no carriage return as on a	195
typewriter.	197
Because the words are typed according to the sound, it	208
is possible to use the machine for recording foreign	219
languages, and the full typewritten translation can be	230
executed by anyone after a minimum of practice in the	241
reading of phonetics in English, and, in the case of	252
other languages, by anyone who understands the language	263
required.	265
One of the main advantages of being able to hand over the	277
typing to others is that the transcribing can be well	288
under way even while the conference meeting is still in	299
progress.	301

The Advantages of the Skill Method

The advantages claimed for this method of teaching are many. First of all, the students always become really interested in what they are doing. In evening classes, where there is often a falling off in attendance after the first few weeks, this is especially noticeable. Where this method has been used, it has been found that attendances are very good throughout the course.

In addition to this, students taught by this method are less tempted to erase or overtype. They have no time to pause to correct errors.

Students trained in this way have been found to be as accurate as those trained by the more traditional methods of teaching typewriting, but it is the author's experience that they reach a very high speed much more quickly. The speed practice loosens the muscles and increases dexterity. It is essential to quick progress and helps the student to type with an even touch.

Teachers will find that this book can be used for day or evening classes. A lesson lasting for more than an hour cannot be used entirely for one-minute timings. During the second half the students can practise on their own. In order to avoid monotony, the teacher can interrupt them from time to time and give them instruction on some point of theory, although by using this book it will be found that students learn a great deal of the theory of typewriting as they go along.

Students of varying degrees of ability can work together. The student who can type at twenty words a minute and the student who can type at eighty words a minute can work at the same time on the same pieces of material, under the same teacher and in the same class, and each can gain the same benefit from the instruction. In fact, the high standard of the quicker students will provide an incentive to the slower ones.

Examinations will seem much less formidable to students who have had their work timed from the first lesson.

The illustration on page 25f has been included to show the teacher how a drill (3b on page 1) is worked. The exercise is typed three times before attempting the one-minute accuracy timing (in many classes twice is sufficient). The sentence is then typed for one minute accurately. In the example, one mistake is made - the student therefore writes "1" in the margin and then notes her speed - in this case 12. The speed timings follow - in each case the student writes down her speed in the margin. Lastly, there is the final one-minute accuracy timing - with a speed of 18 and "0" errors.

A tired old man, clean but in very ragged clothes, was   11
sitting at the side of the road playing a violin, while   22
his little dog held his cap between his teeth for   32
passers-by to throw in their contributions. But the old   43
man knew only a few tunes and even these he could not play   55
well. His bow scraped the strings, making squeaky noises,   67
and the melodies were out of tune. People just gave a   78
quick glance as they passed, and turned away without   89
putting their hands in their pockets for a coin. The   100
poor chap, realizing that it was getting dark and that   111
most pedestrians had gone home, looked at the empty cap   122
and, thinking that no-one would see him, covered his face   134
with his hands and burst into tears.   141
A man had been standing a little distance away, watching   152
him. He came over and said: "May I borrow your violin   163
for a moment please?" He then began to play the most   174
beautiful music and it was not long before many people   185
came, as it seemed, from nowhere, standing in charmed   196
silence as the sounds changed from spring-like dances   207
to the melancholy tunes of loneliness and grief. When   218
the music stopped they all came forward and a shower of   229
silver and notes fell into the old man's cap, and over-   240
flowed on to the road in a great heap. Then the musician   252
played the national anthem, returned the violin to its   263
owner and walked away.   268
No-one knew who he was or where he had come from, but it   279
had been a red-letter day for the old man, who would   290
always remember his kindness.   296

Do not start to type any of the exercises in this book until your teacher tells you how they should be done, or until you have read the instructions at the back of the book for yourself.

All drills are in pica type. If your machine has elite type the letters will appear smaller than the examples in the drills, but follow all instructions as for pica type. Later, from page 34 onwards, you will be given instructions especially for elite type.

The left-hand margin stop should be set at 30. The line-space lever should be set for single-line spacing.

Place your fingers on the home keys (your teacher will show you how to do this). Then memorize the letters shown on the diagram below by repeating them aloud, at the same time making the finger movements necessary for striking the keys ED RF TG YH UJ IK

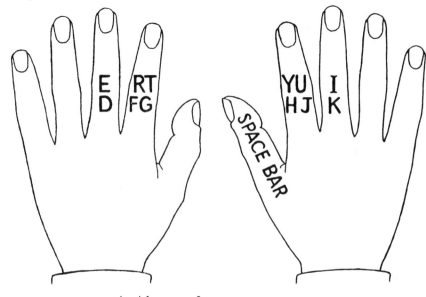

DRILL 1	a.	get the red rug	3
	b.	try the fur rug	3
	c.	they did try it	3
DRILL 2	a.	they did get the key	4
	b.	their key did fit it	4
	c.	hide the fudge there	4
DRILL 3	a.	the judge did fry the egg	5
	b.	they tried the kite there	5
	c.	he did get the free fruit	5

See page 43 for more practice on these letters.

Additional Copying Tests

For pages 50 - 53, set the left-hand margin at 10 for pica, 12 for elite, and the line-space lever for single-line spacing.

DRILL 151

We thank you for your enquiry about our sewing machines.	11
We wish to point out to you that, although you are	21
particularly interested in a hand-operated one, an	31
electric machine would be well worth the extra cost. It	42
is easy to manipulate, is far less tiring for the operator,	54
and garments are produced much more quickly. You may have	66
a demonstration of both types of machine in our showroom	77
at any time, or, if you prefer, we shall be pleased to	88
send a representative to demonstrate to you in your own	99
home. Should you wish to purchase a new machine, we are	110
prepared to take your old one in part exchange and we can	122
also arrange hire-purchase terms if you wish.	131

DRILL 152

As one views Jerusalem from the Mount of Olives, one	11
building stands out prominently from all the rest. This	22
is because of its great golden dome which shines	32
brilliantly in the very hot sun. This vast golden dome	43
surmounts a Moslem mosque which is called the "Dome of the	55
Rock" because it is built over the sacrificial rock of the	67
old Temple of Jerusalem. The mosque stands in the Temple	79
precincts. The Temple precincts consist of a large area	90
of stone-flagged ground where the Great Temple of	100
Solomon once stood, until its destruction in 586 BC.	111
The mosque is perhaps one of the most perfect in the	122
world. It is covered inside and out with the most	132
beautiful mosaics - outside predominantly blue, inside	143
each section of a different design and colour combination.	155
As with all mosques, the floor is covered with hundreds	166
of Persian carpets.	170

Set the left-hand margin stop at 30. Set the line-space lever for single-line spacing.

Type once through the sentences on page 1 (four minutes or less).

Memorize the letters shown on the diagram below by repeating them aloud, at the same time making the finger movements necessary for striking the keys ED RFV TGB YHN UJM IK

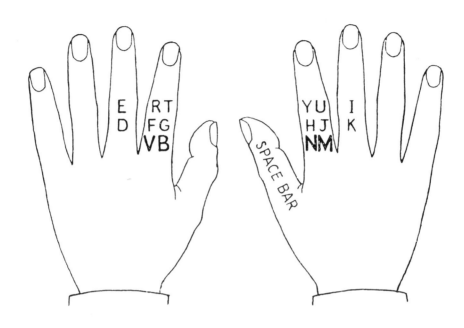

DRILL 4	a.	mend the fender	3
	b.	grind the knife	3
	c.	buy her the gem	3
	d.	buy him the fig	3

DRILL 5	a.	bring them the fruit	4
	b.	feed five hungry men	4
	c.	bring the guide here	4
	d.	mind my big red bike	4

DRILL 6	a.	the men mended the fridge	5
	b.	find my bright green kite	5
	c.	the men did frighten them	5
	d.	they did buy her the mink	5

See page 43 for more practice on these letters.

Spelling at Speed!!

DRILL 146 *(standard words)*

Fulfil, recognize, separate, collated, precise, parallel,
memoirs, wharf, length, foreign, choir, platen, X-rays,
surprise, chief. **(15 words)**

DRILL 147

Restaurant, discipline, protein, pica, fulfilled, occasion,
rhubarb, paradox, contingency, protocol, negotiate, lieutenant,
referred, vandalism, sombre, intercept, precede, equipped,
receive, access. **(20 words)**

DRILL 148

Belief, quorum, recommend, bureau, receipt, debris, transferred,
schedule, February, courtesy, dossier, prestige, courier,
particularly, yacht, recipient, maintenance, definite, bankrupt,
negotiation, occasionally, solemn, accommodation, triumph,
maximum. **(25 words)**

DRILL 149

Courteous, silhouette, residence, upholstery, minimum,
remittance, physician, accommodate, ballet, ascertain,
representative, connoisseur, liaison, embarrass, temporary,
catarrh, piquante, rhythm, fulfilling, colloquial, decision,
pamphlet, exercised, secretary, experience, grammar, quit,
quitted, requirements, referred. **(30 words)**

DRILL 150

Precede, endorsement, brochure, repetition, amateur, elite,
circular, advertisement, centre, extraordinary, grateful,
formula, formulae, regularly, correspondence, column, enquiry,
beginning, mortgage, prompt, adjoining, committee, answer,
friend, gorgeous, hasten, facilities, congested, overhaul,
leisure, alignment, contemporary, luxury, occasionally, column.
(35 words)

Set left-hand margin stop at 30, and the line-space lever for single-line spacing.

Type once through the sentences on page 2 (four minutes or less).

Memorize the letters shown on the diagram below by repeating them aloud, at the same time making the finger movements necessary for striking the keys EDC RFV TGB YHN UJM IK,

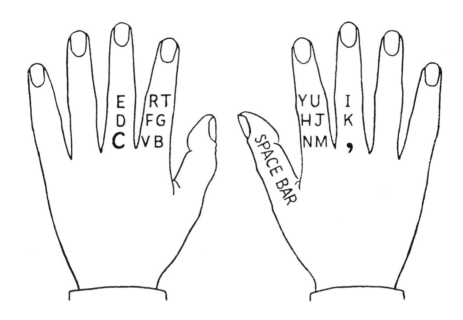

DRILL 7	a.	mum hid the gun	3
	b.	he hit her chin	3
	c.	chide the guide	3
	d.	buy the red jug	3

DRILL 8	a.	he did the big trick	4
	b.	the judge did cringe	4
	c.	give him the big tin	4
	d.	he might buy the net	4

DRILL 9	a.	bring me the bigger cruet	5
	b.	in time, he might give in	5
	c.	nine men tried, then five	5
	d.	try the fried minced beef	5

See page 44 for more practice on these letters.

Roman Numerals

DRILL 144

The capitals letters O, I, V, X, L, C, D, M, are used for Roman numerals. These stand for 0, 1, 5, 10, 50, 100, 500, 1000.

Two or three of the same letters may be used together, i.e. XX, XXX, CC, CCC, MM, MMM, which represent 20, 30, 200, 300, 2,000, 3,000.

When two numbers of different value are to be added together, the larger number comes first, followed by the smaller, i.e. VI, XII, XXVI, LXX, DL. These stand for 6, 12, 26, 70, 550.

If the smaller number is to be subtracted from the greater it is placed before the larger number, i.e. IV, IX, CM, XL: these read 4, 9, 900, 40.

A line drawn over a Roman numeral multiplies that number by a thousand. C (100), $\overline{C}$ (100,000). M (1,000), $\overline{M}$ (1,000,000), a thousand thousand, or one million. L (50), $\overline{L}$ (50,000).

Numbers containing a figure four or a figure nine must be obtained by subtraction, e.g. CHAPTER IV, George IV, CHAPTER IX, XL, or XC. (Chapter 4, George 4th, Chapter 9, 40, or 90).

Never use 'st', 'nd', or 'th' after Roman numerals.

The lower-case letters i, v, x, etc. are calculated as above, but are normally used for the preliminary pages of a book, or sometimes in lists.

Superior and Inferior Characters

DRILL 145

These are more easily arranged by raising or lowering the line of typing by half a line-space, rather than by using the Variable line spacer, because it is simpler and quicker to return to the original level. When a group of these characters is required type everything on the line of typing first, leaving the necessary spaces for the raised or lowered characters. Then raise or lower the level to insert the extra characters.

EXAMPLE

$$a^2 - b^3 - c^2 d^3 - e^5 - f^2 - g^3 - h^2$$

$$x_2 - y_3 - z_2 - x_4 - y_3 z_2 - x_5 - z_3$$

Set the left-hand margin stop at 30, and the line-space lever for single-line spacing.

Type once through the sentences on page 3 (four minutes or less).

Memorize the letters shown on the diagram below by repeating them aloud, at the same time making the finger movements necessary for striking the keys WSX EDC RFV TGB YHN UJM IK, OL

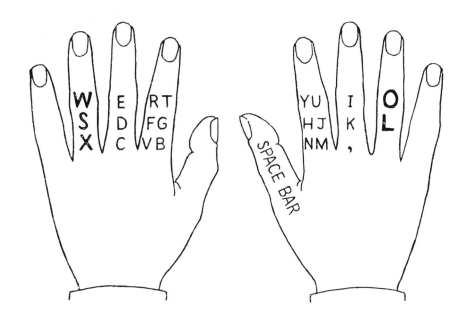

DRILL 10	a.	wind this clock	3
	b.	fetch the goods	3
	c.	close your eyes	3
	d.	mind these boys	3

DRILL 11	a.	fix these six screws	4
	b.	lend her sixty books	4
	c.	they tested the mike	4
	d.	she wore blue denims	4

DRILL 12	a.	churn the butter tomorrow	5
	b.	he enjoyed the fried rice	5
	c.	four young men went there	5
	d.	seven men mixed the dough	5

See page 44 for extra practice on these letters.

Additional Practice - Signs and Accents

DRILL 139	Are they quite sure?	4
	What an awful noise!	4
	<u>Do</u> be quiet, please!	4
	Book seats 4, 5 & 6.	4
DRILL 140	I am twenty-one tomorrow.	5
	Buy seven day-old chicks.	5
	Great Scott! Look there!	5
	"Go to bed", said Mother.	5
DRILL 141	Oh dear! Another traffic jam!	6
	Cheer up! What is the matter?	6
	Tickets Nos 15 & 16 were sold.	6
	Type on <u>one side</u> of the paper.	6
DRILL 142	£1 15s. (old money) is worth £1.75.	7
	"Hey, there! Where are you going?"	7
	That four-year-old child is clever.	7
	Payne, Dodd & Co. are now bankrupt.	7
DRILL 143	Smith & Co. have made 149 men redundant.	8
	The firm gave £16 (8%) discount on £200.	8
	The order was for 4196 books @ 75p each.	8
	A date might sometimes be typed 27/7/79.	8

Accents

Signs or marks which are not represented on a typewriter, can
sometimes be made up by using two others, i.e. ÷ (hyphen with a
colon over it), and the 'equal' sign = by using two hyphens and
lowering the second one by using the variable line spacer.
Accents or any other signs which cannot be represented on the
machine in any way, must be inserted afterwards in ink.

Set the left-hand margin stop at 30, and the line-space lever for single-line spacing.

Type once through the sentences on page 4 (four minutes or less).

Memorize the letters shown on the diagram below by repeating them aloud, at the same time making the finger movements necessary for striking the keys QAZ WSX EDC RFV TGB YHN UJM IK, OL P;

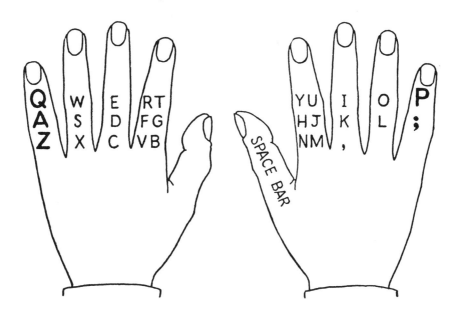

DRILL 13   a.   paint the walls   3

           b.   use the new axe   3

           c.   please be quiet   3

           d.   scrub the floor   3

DRILL 14   a.   come to the big fair   4

           b.   she never told a lie   4

           c.   we went to the party   4

           d.   you can play the sax   4

DRILL 15   a.   be ready for a quick walk   5

           b.   he was young; he was lazy   5

           c.   she won a prize yesterday   5

           d.   squeeze these lemons well   5

See page 45 for extra practice on these letters.

Additional Practice - Numbers

Set the left-hand margin stop at 10, and the line-space lever for single-line spacing. The following counting is in standard words.

DRILL 138

(a)

Denis Clark, aged 26, lives at 97 Sefton Avenue. His girl friend lives at No. 54. They are getting married and are going to live at 138 Oxford Avenue, York.   **(30 words)**

(b)

The winning team scored 278 in the first innings and 296 in the second. The losing team scored 145 and 209. Jack scored 123 and King bowled four for 17.   **(30 words)**

(c)

Kindly send 750 extra large notebooks and 900 small ones, 240 sheets of carbon paper and 250 pencils. Please deliver this order to 67 Crozeley Road, London, N1 6NU. I need these articles immediately.   **(35 words)**

(d)

We chose six of the patterns you sent us and we would like you to forward 24 metres of these materials. The pattern numbers are: J12, 34, V56, 78, Z9 and 10. Please address to 20 Queen Street, Leigh, Staffs.   **(40 words)**

(e)

We are holding our summer sale next week. The most popular items to be reduced are 50 coats, 200 long skirts, 890 dresses, 470 jumpers with zips, and 136 very smart hats. The reductions range from a quarter to a half of the marked prices.   **(45 words)**

(f)

England's beauty queen contest is held annually in a popular holiday resort. The girls parade in swim suits in the public gardens, and later, in a local hall wearing evening gowns. Their ages are usually from 17 to 23 years. Recently, Joan S. came 1st, Betty M. 2nd, Rita D. 3rd, Mary R. 4th and Joanna B. 5th.   **(50 words)**

Set the left-hand margin stop at 30, and the line-space lever for single-line spacing.

Type once through the sentences on page 5 (three minutes or less).

Revise all the letters shown on the diagram below by repeating them aloud, at the same time making the finger movements necessary for striking the keys QAZ WSX EDC RFV TGB YHN UJM IK, OL. P;

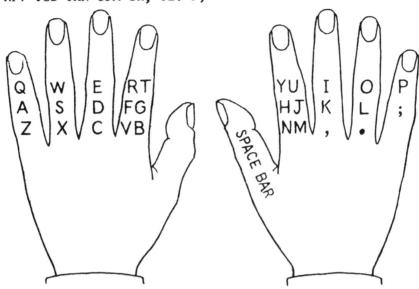

Notice the position of the shift keys on your machine. These keys are used when you wish to strike a capital letter. Use the right-hand shift key for letters struck with the fingers of the left hand, and the left-hand shift key for letters struck with the fingers of the right hand. When you wish to strike a capital letter: (1) Using the little finger strike and <u>hold down</u> the shift key. (2) Strike the required key. (3) Release the shift key.

DRILL 16	a.	The bee buzzes.	3
	b.	Fetch his coat.	3
	c.	Play that game.	3
	d.	Have some fizz.	3
DRILL 17	a.	Fix your seat belts.	4
	b.	Pray for a fine day.	4
	c.	Ice my cake quickly.	4
	d.	Check all your work.	4
DRILL 18	a.	Those flowers need water.	5
	b.	I need a red baize cloth.	5
	c.	Put the seeds in the box.	5
	d.	Buy some more new tights.	5

See page 45 for extra practice on capital letters.

DRILL 136
for Page 5

```
Q   W   E   RT  YU   I   O   P
A   S   D   FG  HJ   K   L   ;
Z   X   C   VB  NM       ,
```

women claim equal pay with men   6

play that sax in the jazz band   6

she goes to the city every day   6

she is neat, tidy and reliable   6

they saw two zebras at the zoo   6

that honey cost a lot of money   6

she wrote books; he wrote odes   6

she played the harp quite well   6

wash these thirty dirty shirts   6

she finished the quilt quickly   6

DRILL 137
for Page 6

```
Q   W   E   RT  YU   I   O   P
A   S   D   FG  HJ   K   L   ;
```
Shift   `Z   X   C   VB  NM   ,   .`   Shift
key   key

You should get an Access card.   6

Do not exceed the speed limit.   6

Cover the chairs with draylon.   6

He wants to be a jazz pianist.   6

Put crazy paving on the patio.   6

Matthew used my new car today.   6

I need six extra large plates.   6

Sit quite quietly for a while.   6

Join us for a walk on Tuesday.   6

Fire the machine gun; now run.   6

Set the left-hand margin stop at 30, and the line-space lever for single-line spacing.

DRILL 19 a. I like to read in the evenings. 6

b. Come to the bank with me today. 6

c. Forward the black pens quickly. 6

d. Kindly give me a ring tomorrow. 6

e. Robert bought six jazz records. 6

Set the left-hand margin stop at 20, and the line-space lever for double-line spacing. Follow the line-endings given below, returning the carriage at the end of each line.

Leave *two* spaces after a full stop at the end of a sentence.

DRILL 20

Please send us sixty pairs of black shoes for women, 11

size seven, as advertised in your catalogue on page 21

twelve. They appear to be just what we require and 31

they are of very good value. 37

DRILL 21

Some envelopes have panels in the front which are 10

either left open or covered with transparent paper. 20

Letters are then folded and inserted in them so that 31

the address is visible through the panel. 39

DRILL 22

The junior razors we ordered arrived today and we 10

now enclose a cheque in payment of the account. Will 21

you kindly forward ten boxes of blades, as we quite 31

forgot to order these at the same time. 39

DRILL 134
for Page 3

```
E   RT  YU  I
D   FG  HJ  K
C   VB  NM  ,
```

they met her by the beech tree   6

give them drink in the big jug   6

the mimic mimicked the ten men   6

the three men died in the fire   6

thirteen men run, five give in   6

nine men tried the fire engine   6

they fetched the bike by truck   6

the men trimmed the high hedge   6

he did buy her the nutty fudge   6

get the men to mend the gutter   6

DRILL 135
for Page 4

```
W   E   RT  YU  I   O
S   D   FG  HJ  K   L
X   C   VB  NM  ,
```

give the green ties to the boy   6

this nice yellow dress is mine   6

the birds nested in the shrubs   6

weigh the fudge in the kitchen   6

show him the route to the club   6

fix the hinge on the side door   6

do the work from the next text   6

he mended it, it is just right   6

she wore nice new white tights   6

men or women do these big jobs   6

Set the left-hand margin stop at 30, and the line-space lever for single-line spacing.

DRILL 23 a.   He saw the train enter the station.   **7**

           b.   The jugs have arrived quite safely.   **7**

           c.   Black dogs won prizes at the shows.   **7**

           d.   The box is old and is worth little.   **7**

           e.   Please send him a copy of the book.   **7**

Set the left-hand margin stop at 20, and the line-space lever for double-line spacing. Follow the line-endings given below.

Remember to leave *two* spaces after a full stop at the end of a sentence.

DRILL 24

     Our office is small but it is well equipped. It has   **11**

     a telephone, several filing cabinets and six chairs   **21**

     and desks. We work zealously for a good firm, and the   **32**

     manager has just said that we are to have a rise.   **42**

DRILL 25

     A mace was originally used in battle and was carried   **10**

     by a clergyman instead of a sword. The present one in   **21**

     the House of Commons is over three hundred years old.   **32**

     It is the symbol of the authority of the Speaker.   **42**

DRILL 26

     We are sorry to have to complain about the quality of   **11**

     the jade cardigans. We needed extra thick ones with   **22**

     zip fasteners instead of buttons. Will you send this   **32**

     type of cardigan in place of these which we will   **42**

     return.   **43**

Additional Practice

DRILL 132
for Page 1

```
E   RT   YU   I
D   FG   HJ   K
```

they did try the red kite here   6

he did get the right gift here   6

the red tug drifted fifty feet   6

the grit hurt their tired feet   6

the rugged digger dug the dyke   6

the judge did get her the gift   6

feed the grey furry kitty here   6

hide the hefty key right there   6

they did get the jute rug dyed   6

he did hide the huge red fruit   6

DRILL 133
for Page 2

```
E   RT   YU   I
D   FG   HJ   K
    VB   NM
```

he did bring the king the ring   6

the men did hurry by the ferry   6

he mended the bunk in the junk   6

he did regret the thing he did   6

did the fire burn the five men   6

did he find the kinky mink fur   6

bring the ginger beer jug here   6

judge the red beet in the fete   6

the men mended the bent fender   6

bring him the bright green mug   6

Set the left-hand margin stop at 28, and the line-space lever for single-line spacing.

DRILL 27
a. It was kind of you to answer my letters.   8

b. Johnny hopes to hear from you next week.   8

c. It will be a pleasure to see your agent.   8

d. I require a very large baize tablecloth.   8

e. The new secretary waited for her salary.   8

Set the left-hand margin stop at 20, and the line-space lever for double-line spacing. Remember to leave *two* spaces after a full stop at the end of a sentence.

DRILL 28

The men at the quarry are expected to work for seven   11

hours a day; sometimes they do overtime to earn more   21

money. They get just a little more each hour if they   32

work after five, but they are usually lazy at this   42

time.   43

DRILL 29

The Post Office recommends that envelopes of only   10

certain sizes should be used so that they can be sorted   21

in the modern electronic equipment. These are known as   32

POP envelopes and the initials stand for Post Office   43

Preferred.   45

DRILL 30

The yellow pages of a telephone directory, which are   11

now published as a separate book, classify trades and   22

professions. These are given in alphabetical order   32

under such headings as Builders, Restaurants, Schools,   43

Handicrafts and so on.   47

Set the left-hand margin stop at 20, and the line-space lever for single-line spacing.

```
DRILL 129        (a)    east earn eddy enjoy                           4
  E and I               else cake rote crude                          4

                        ibex icon idle ideal                          4
                        quit grid snip print                          4

                        pies tied diet quiet                          4
                        vein leis weir deity                          4

          (b)    dies pied replied belief believe pierrot             8
                 piece pierce pier piety sobriety friends             8
                 receive conceived deceit ceiling veiling             8
                 extinct exits exquisite extensive fiends             8


DRILL 130        (a)    fluid fruit suitable                          4
 UI and IU              acquit quire acquire                          4

                        helium genius barium                          4
                        calcium valium opium                          4

                        liquid union quietly                          4
                        requite sequin guilt                          4

          (b)    precious guise dubious gymnasium furious             8
                 fortuitous emporium curious envious lieu             8
                 suits magnesium symposium union cautious             8
                 solarium tenacious pretentious fractious             8


DRILL 131        (a)    comb came chip cramp                          4
  C and V               nice brac chic trace                          4

                        vein vane vile vogue                          4
                        dove five gave shove                          4

                        cave cove vice vocal                          4
                        voices civil voucher                          4

          (b)    groves vortex covetous craving voracious             8
                 convey victim vacuum avocado controversy             8
                 vicarage convoy convent viceroy vocalist             8
                 convener concave viking crevasse vacancy             8
```

Set the left-hand margin stop at 25, and the line-space lever for single-line spacing.

Notice the position of the *question mark* on your machine, and use the appropriate finger.

DRILL 31

a.	Did the boy enjoy the play on the television?	9
b.	Did you put the books in the safe last night?	9
c.	What is the total cost of production to date?	9
d.	Where will you go for your holiday next year?	9
e.	How many queries have you settled this month?	9

Set the left-hand margin stop at 20, and the line-space lever for single-line spacing.

DRILL 32

A quarter of the number of zinc buckets you sent were	11
damaged in transit. This is annoying, and we are all	22
the more vexed because it is only just a year since	32
we started dealing with you, and we keep having to	42
complain of careless packing.	48

DRILL 33

Big Ben is, I understand, the largest clock in the	10
world, although from the ground one would not think so.	21
The figures are two feet long and the dials measure	31
nearly eighty feet across. The ornamental work on the	42
clock was designed by Pugin.	48

DRILL 34

We need five more men in this zone to help us with the	11
extra work and unless you can send them along the job	22
cannot be finished in time. We quite realize that you	33
cannot easily spare them from other work, but in this	44
case it is essential.	48

Set the left-hand margin stop at 20, and the line-space lever for single-line spacing.

DRILL 126   (a)   upon undo user ulcer   4
  U and Y   true clue flue queue   4

                          yard yoke year yeast   4
                          wily very holy merry   4

                          fury duty puny young   4
                          ruby buoy jury youth   4

         (b)   utility youth thundery yuletide beautify   8

                curry mutiny yoghurt cutlery gully baudy   8

                joyful guilty popularity butterfly rusty   8

                curly yellow crucify yourself unity ugly   8

DRILL 127   (a)   jute jazz jest jewel   4
  J and H   jowl jump junk jetty   4

                          hire home heap hovel   4
                          rash both kith peach   4

                          joss sash jilt heath   4
                          hate jeer jade jingo   4

         (b)   thrifty thermal heather theology thimble   8

                heirloom ahead phenomenon honour heights   8

                justice adjacent jocular eject adjoining   8

                adjunct jester joyful rejoice rejuvenate   8

DRILL 128   (a)   mite move maul marry   4
  M and N   maim boom team theme   4

                          nape need newt north   4
                          vane boon gain shunt   4

                          mint mine numb enemy   4
                          mien moan amen money   4

         (b)   coalman namesake normal demons tramlines   8

                anemone mundane morning undermine tandem   8

                pomander mnemonic famine minstrel mantra   8

                unmanned nutriment managing miners money   8

Set the left-hand margin stop at 20, and the line-space lever for single-line spacing.

DRILL 35

a.   We thank you very much for your letter of yesterday.   10

b.   We have a large assortment of jumpers and cardigans.   10

c.   They did the job twice but it was not quite correct.   10

d.   The big box kites should fly high in the wind today.   10

e.   Please send samples of your small wallets with zips.   10

Set the left-hand margin stop at 20, and the line-space lever for single-line spacing.

DRILL 36

The lease on the office on the sixth floor comes to an   11
end on the last day of the year. It will thus be   21
necessary for us to move fairly quickly to new premises   32
in a different zone, and we have just decided that this   43
would be quite a good time for us to expand.   52

DRILL 37

Spend a very pleasant day in a narrow boat on the   10
Regents Canal, known as Little Venice. The scenery is   21
a mixture of derelict buildings, green banks and trees,   32
and fine old houses. The boat also passes the aviary   43
at the Zoo which was designed by Lord Snowdon.   52

DRILL 38

Children should be taught rules of road safety at a   10
very early age by their parents, and by their teachers   21
when they are old enough to join a class. Parents and   32
teachers must be zealous in showing how necessary it is   43
to think quickly and to cross the road carefully.   52

Common Error Drills

Set the left-hand margin stop at 20, and the line-space lever for single-line spacing.

DRILL 123 R and T	(a)	road race rice reach	4
		door pear four spear	4
		tyre trap trim track	4
		part hurt dirt sport	4
		tier raft root their	4
		trot rate tart treat	4
	(b)	revert concert divert alert overt insert	8
		turnip concrete contradict tramp replete	8
		repeat temperate hydrant biretta trumpet	8
		matter fitter otter mutter setter hooter	8
DRILL 124 F and G	(a)	fall find from flues	4
		buff chef waif scarf	4
		good grey gone green	4
		bang plug slog prong	4
		flag gulf fags grief	4
		gaff figs flog fungi	4
	(b)	fright gratify fatigue profligate gruffy	8
		fridge fatigue flogging fragile giraffes	8
		magnificent frugal refrigerator grateful	8
		grief effigy flagrantly fungicide fringe	8
DRILL 125 V and B	(a)	vine vane vole verse	4
		love give move mauve	4
		bite boar buck blaze	4
		daub crib slub shrub	4
		verb value vestibule	4
		bevy above available	4
	(b)	obvious beloved variable believe bravery	8
		vibrant vegetables verbal vagabond bravo	8
		venerable viable beavers vibrates bovril	8
		oblivion observatory absolves abbreviate	8

Set the left-hand margin stop at 20, and the line-space lever for single-line spacing.

DRILL 39

a.   We will forward your boxes by rail on Thursday morning.   **11**

b.   The shop is shut today for the purpose of taking stock.   **11**

c.   We have quite a large number of school blazers on sale.   **11**

d.   The silk is just a shade darker than the red we wanted.   **11**

e.   We hope to hear from them in the course of a few weeks.   **11**

Set the left-hand margin stop at 20, and the line-space lever for single-line spacing.

DRILL 40

    We regret that we cannot extend the time of reduced   **10**
    prices, as the offer was popular this year and our   **20**
    stocks were completely sold out within the month. In **31**
    view of this, shall we cancel your order or would you **42**
    prefer that we send the goods and you forward the   **52**
    balance?   **54**

DRILL 41

    In order to obtain perfect evenness of touch when   **10**
    typing, punctuation marks should be struck with less   **21**
    force than the other keys, or they will pierce the   **31**
    paper and leave a roughness at the back. On the other **42**
    hand, capital letters should be given slightly more   **52**
    pressure.   **54**

DRILL 42

    Football is probably the most popular game in this   **10**
    country. Matches are held every weekend during the   **21**
    season in most towns of any size, and also at midweek. **32**
    As the midweek matches are normally evening matches   **42**
    grounds are equipped with special lighting. Matches   **52**
    are enjoyed by thousands.   **57**

DRILL 121 (a)

Typewriters have been in general use for over 100 years. Some of	13
the first models were very ornate and the paintings on them must have	26
been quite distracting to a typist. Apart from this, the keys when	40
struck, made more noise than the modern ones, and the work typed could	54
not be seen without lifting the carriage. Instead of ribbons there	67
were inked pads, and on some models there were two sets of keys for the	81
alphabet - one for lower-case letters and the other above it for capital	96
letters.	98

DRILL 121 (b)

A backing sheet, which is a piece of stiff paper used behind the	12
page on which you type, is useful for many purposes. It helps to give	26
a more even impression to the work and prevents the back of the docu-	40
ment from showing the marks of the keys. It also prevents some wear	54
and tear on the platen surface. If a thick line in black is drawn on	68
it about two inches from the bottom, it shows through the paper	80
sufficiently to indicate that you can type only one or two more lines	94
on that page. Always use a backing sheet.	102

DRILL 122 (a)

It is very necessary at this stage in the expansion of our business	13
to determine whether we shall confine our activities to the British	26
Isles, or whether we shall attempt to find other markets for our	39
goods in the countries of E.E.C. (European Economic Community). I	52
feel sure that these markets exist, but it will mean sending our	66
representatives who speak the languages of these countries to contact	79
their buyers in order to procure substantial export orders.	93
	105

DRILL 122 (b)

Every typist should understand how the ribbon mechanism works on	12
the machine she uses, and she should be able to insert a new ribbon	26
when the old one is worn out. It is a simple process. Wind the old	39
ribbon on to the right-hand spool, remove it from the machine, and	52
insert the new spool in its place. Attach the end of the new ribbon	68
to the empty left-hand spool and place it in position. Before re-	81
moving the worn ribbon, notice how it is slotted into the ribbon	94
vibrator, because this varies with different makes of typewriter.	105

Set the left-hand margin stop at 28, and the line-space lever for single-line spacing.

Use a small "el" for the *figure 1* if your machine is not fitted with a special key for this character.

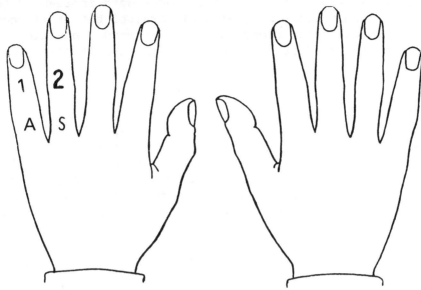

DRILL 43 a. There were 111 men working on the ships.   8

b. On Thursday 11 children passed the test.   8

c. There are 212 people at the whist drive.   8

d. The bus crashed and 12 men were injured.   8

e. There were 212 boys, but only 112 girls.   8

Set the left-hand margin stop at 15 (pica), 18 (elite), and the line-space lever for single-line spacing.

Notice the positions of the *tabulator key* or bar, and of the tabulator set key, on your machine. Use the tabulator for the indentation at the beginning of paragraphs. To set the tabulator, move the carriage to the left-hand margin, strike the space bar five times for pica and six for elite (half inch), and then press the tabulator set key. To indent the first line of a paragraph, move the carriage to the left-hand margin, and then strike and hold down the tabulator key or bar until the carriage has moved to the required position.

DRILL 44

It is the duty of the firm to pay the men if they work.   11

DRILL 45

We must work well always if we wish to reach the   10
top, for without hard work success is very seldom   20
obtained. It is of little use to work only on days   30
when we feel inclined to do so, so we must go on each   41
day, with zeal, to the end.   46

DRILL 119 (a)

Given that there is a half-space bar on your machine, and you wish   13
to erase a word to replace it with one containing an extra letter, just   27
leave a half space before and after the longer word instead of the usual   41
whole one. The result looks very slightly cramped but it is accept-   55
able. For the reverse situation, to replace a word containing one   70
letter less than the word erased, leave one-and-a-half spaces on each   84
side of it.   86

DRILL 119 (b)

Figures or letters which are typed slightly above or below the line   13
of typing are called superior and inferior characters respectively.   26
They are placed in these positions by moving the platen very slightly   38
up or down, by the use of the variable line spacer which, on modern   52
machines, is depressed while the platen is moved into the required   65
place. Superior and inferior characters are used in chemical and   79
algebraic formulae, or as references to footnotes.   89

DRILL 120 (a)

Legal and technical documents such as Specifications and Bills of   13
Quantities are folded in four, approximately to the size of a foolscap   27
envelope, and are then endorsed. An endorsement contains the date at   40
the top (across the narrow width), the name of the document about 2½ ins   55
lower down (usually in spaced capitals), then 2½ ins or so further down,   69
the name(s) of the partners in the document. Lastly, at the bottom,   83
the name and address of the firm, i.e. of the lawyer or builder.   96

DRILL 120 (b)

Headings are usually typed in capitals, but if there are two, the   13
more important one should be in spaced capitals, that is, there should   27
be one space after every letter in the heading, and three spaces between   41
the words. The second heading should be in closed capitals - no spaces   55
between the letters, but two spaces between the words. Leave at least   69
one inch at the top of the paper, and three line spaces between the   83
headings. Sometimes it is more effective _not_ to underline them.   96

Set the left-hand margin stop at 28, and the line-space lever for single-line spacing.

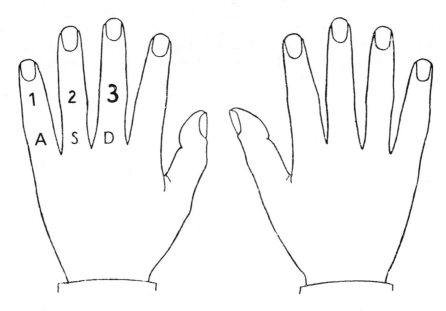

DRILL 46 a. The school had 333 children on the roll.   8

          b. One teacher had 32 infants in her class.   8

          c. Six times a week 11 girls went swimming.   8

          d. The other 21 asked to learn audiotyping.   8

          e. There were only 3 typewriters available.   8

Set the left-hand margin stop at 15, and the line-space lever for single-line spacing.

DRILL 47

    The maid may mend socks for them if she is paid for it.   11

DRILL 48

        The full stop, besides being used at the end of a   10
    sentence, is used for the decimal point, after initials   21
    and abbreviations, and for leader dots in tabulations.   32
    It is only at the end of a sentence, however, that two   43
    spaces are left after it.   48

DRILL 116 (b)

Please type memos to each department asking members of the staff	12
to cut down the number of personal telephone calls they make during	26
office hours. Also point out that, although the Office Manager has no	39
objection to the occasional use of the telephone for private calls,	53
they should not be allowed to become so frequent as to interfere with	66
the efficient working of the switchboard.	75

DRILL 117 (a)

Typewriting speeds are calculated in two ways - by counting in	12
five-stroke words, or by using standard words. The latter just means	26
counting the actual number of words typed, regardless of length. For	39
the former method, all the letters, spaces and punctuation marks must	53
be totalled and the result divided by five. In each case, the number	67
obtained is divided by the number of minutes taken.	77

DRILL 117 (b)

Although there are two systems used to assess typing speed, the	12
five-stroke word method and the standard method, the first gives a	25
slightly higher result than the second. However, as it is calculated	39
on every depression of the keys made by the typist compared with the	52
actual number of words of whatever length as in the second method, it	66
is perhaps a fairer way of estimating speed.	77

DRILL 118 (a)

If you are an accurate typist you will seldom need to erase, but,	13
when it is necessary, it should be done with care. Move the carriage	26
to the extreme left or right, so that dust from the eraser falls out-	40
side the machine, and then erase gently. Errors on carbon copies must	57
be erased separately. A great deal of time is lost, however, by	67
erasing, so type as quickly as you can without making errors.	79

DRILL 118 (b)

Some machines have a second, shorter space bar alongside the main	13
one, which, when it is depressed, moves the carriage along only half	26
a space instead of the usual whole one. This space bar can be used	40
when material is required to be typed with a straight right-hand margin.	54
Another use for it is the correction of errors when replacing a word of	68
one more, or one less the number of letters than the incorrect word	82
which has been erased.	86

Set the left-hand margin stop at 28, and the line-space lever for single-line spacing.

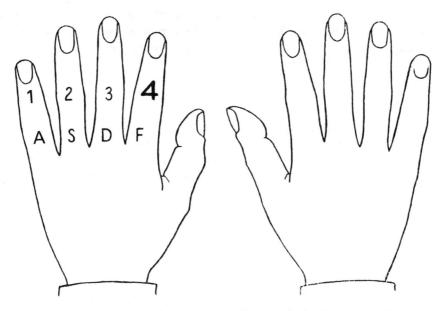

DRILL 49 a.   Their scores yesterday were 113 and 114.   8

          b.   The tennis match was played on 14th May.   8

          c.   The library bought 412 books this month.   8

          d.   I bought 14 litre bottles of white wine.   8

          e.   12 x 12 makes 144; this is just a gross.   8

Set the left-hand margin stop at 15, and the line-space lever for single-line spacing.

DRILL 50

    They make cocoa for the men when they work by the dock.   11

DRILL 51

        Please send, by return if possible, four dozen   9
fountain pens to be used for shorthand writing in our   20
College. We prefer the fine nibs, and, if there is a   31
choice of colour, please let us have a dozen of each   42
shade, including a dozen black ones.   48

DRILL 114 (a)

Before cutting a stencil see that the type is clean. Then move	12
the ribbon lever to the stencil position which is usually marked by a	26
white line or dot. Place a sheet of carbon paper between the stencil	40
and the backing sheet, with the carbon surface towards the stencil.	53
Type with a firm, even touch.	59

DRILL 114 (b)

Chain feeding saves a good deal of time when cards and envelopes	12
are required to be typed. This simply means that the next card or	26
envelope to be typed is inserted before the finished one is moved. One	40
movement of the platen releases the completed card, and, at the same	53
time, brings the next one into its position for typing.	64

DRILL 115 (a)

Teletourist is a branch of the Telephone Information Service which	13
will give details of the events of the day taking place in and around	27
London. There are separate numbers in the telephone directory which	40
you can ring for this information according to whether you wish to	53
obtain an answer in English, French, German, Spanish or Italian.	66

DRILL 115 (b)

The art of typing material with a straight right-hand margin is not	13
often required and can only be done on a machine with a special es-	26
capement. This produces a "justified" right-hand margin. It is some-	39
what complicated at first because a number of calculations have to be	53
made for each page, but it is explained fully in a good dictionary of	66
typewriting.	68

DRILL 116 (a)

Skill in typewriting can be acquired only by regular and concen-	13
trated practice. It is necessary to type a great number of repetitive	27
sentences - daily if possible - and to copy a large amount of straight-	40
forward matter accurately and quickly. High speed in shorthand is	55
useless if the notes cannot be transcribed reasonably quickly on the	69
typewriter.	71

Set the left-hand margin stop at 28, and the line-space lever for single-line spacing.

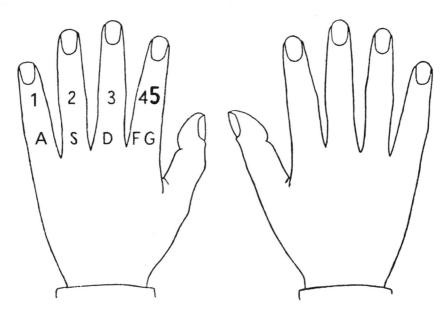

DRILL 52 a.   There are 31 days in March and December.   8

           b.   Please send 35 sacks of logs on Tuesday.   8

           c.   The assistants sold 145 m of blue satin.   8

           d.   We ordered 55 items but he sent only 15.   8

           e.   11 x 11 makes 121 and 15 x 15 makes 225.   8

Set the left-hand margin stop at 15, and the line-space lever for single-line spacing.

DRILL 53

   Turn to the right by the big sign to go to the field.   11

DRILL 54

     We can now supply you with the goods ordered last   10
month. Six dozen scarves will be sent off today, and   21
the rest at the end of the week. We regret that we are   32
still unable to supply the berets in all the colours you   43
wanted, but these will be sent later.   50

Set the margin stops so that the margins on the left and right are both 1½ inches wide (or 40 mm), line-space lever for single-line spacing.

Remember to listen for the bell, and keep your right-hand margin as even as possible.

DRILL 111 (a)

Ghost or shadow letters on a page of typing are caused by	11
the operator lingering on the keys when striking them. Keys	23
must be struck sharply in order that the type bars will move quickly	37
away from the printing point.	43

DRILL 111 (b)

An excellent practice is to type straight on to the typewriter from	13
dictation or from recordings made on discs or tapes. Machines on	26
which recordings are made are called audio machines: if you learn	40
to use them you can become an audio typist.	48

DRILL 112 (a)

The man took up his stand at the end of the almost derelict jetty	13
and thought of how the years of exile were telling upon him. He had	26
found plenty of occupation at the beginning of his life on the island,	40
but, as the years passed, he had become lazy.	50

DRILL 112 (b)

An abacus is a simple visual aid for obtaining the answers to	12
addition, subtraction, multiplication and division of numbers, using	25
the denary and other systems of counting. The denary system is that	39
of counting in units, tens, hundreds, thousands, etc.	50

DRILL 113 (a)

We have seen that the system of calculating in tens is called the	13
denary system. Some other systems are the binary, counting in twos,	26
seximal, counting in sixes, and octal, counting in eights. The binary	40
system is that used for electronic digital computer programming.	53

DRILL 113 (b)

The velvet curtains which one of your men fixed last week are not	13
quite satisfactory. The hooks do not slide along easily and they	26
appear to be unevenly arranged. If you will kindly ask him to call	39
again, I am sure that a small adjustment will put the matter right.	53

Set the left-hand margin stop at 28, and the line-space lever for single-line spacing.

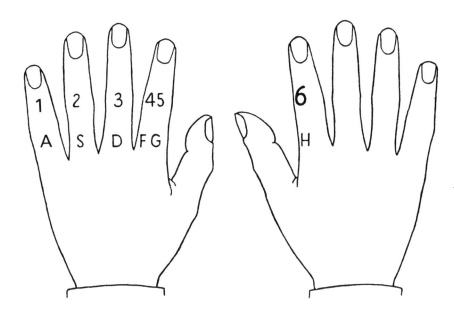

DRILL 55 a. He lives at 6 Avons, Birmingham B16 5TS.   8

          b. A tour has been arranged for 156 people.   8

          c. 24, 36 and 144 are each divisible by 12.   8

          d. Kindly send 66 safety razors on Tuesday.   8

          e. This bus company put on 166 extra buses.   8

Set the left-hand margin stop at 15, and the line-space lever for single-line spacing.

DRILL 56

    The eight girls may wish to go with them to the city.   11

DRILL 57

        With regard to the eight empty boxes which you say   10
    were forwarded to us on Tuesday, we regret to say that   21
    we cannot trace having received these. Will you kindly   32
    ask the carriers to prove delivery, otherwise we shall   43
    be obliged to charge the cases to your account.   52

Set the margin stops so that the margins on the left and right are *both* 1½ inches wide (or 40 mm). To do this correctly you must, first of all, notice the size of the type on the machine you are using. If it is the same size as the exercise at the beginning of this book, it is called **pica** type and this measures 10 letters to the inch. If it is **elite** type, it measures 12 letters to the inch. Therefore set the margins at 15 and 67 for **pica** type, and at 18 and 82 for **elite** type.

A4 sheets contain 82 letters across the page in **pica** type and 100 letters across the page in **elite** type.

In the following exercises, which are in a smaller type, you must make your own right-hand margin, returning the carriage after the bell rings. If necessary, divide words by using a hyphen at the line-ending. Your teacher will tell you how to do this. The line-space lever should be set for single-line spacing.

DRILL 108 (a)

The duplicator in the office is a very old one. It is soon	11
being replaced by a more expensive new model in the new year.	24

DRILL 108 (b)

The increase in the number of customers in this new area has	12
exceeded our hopes, and because of this, we may need extra regular	25
supplies.	27

DRILL 109 (a)

Kindly despatch, as soon as possible, sixty umbrellas as adver-	12
tised on page three of your catalogue. Owing to the wet weather	25
sales have been heavy and our stock is low.	34

DRILL 109 (b)

Computers are basically electronic calculators. They can also	12
store information which can be added to or altered, and this is fed	25
into the machine in the form of coded numbers.	34

DRILL 110 (a)

It is surprising how with a little thought one can avoid the	12
division of a word at the end of a line, and it is seldom necessary	25
unless the word has at least three syllables.	34

DRILL 110 (b)

An abacus is a counting frame consisting of a small, flat, oblong	13
board in which several holes are bored to hold stiff wires on which	26
beads or discs can be placed to act as counters.	36

Set the left-hand margin stop at 28, and the line-space lever for single-line spacing.

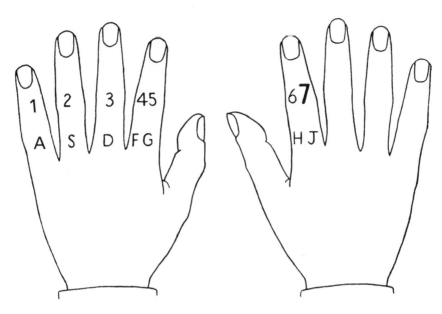

DRILL 58   a.   Out of 117 baskets of fruit 17 were bad.   8

           b.   There were 147 ships in port on Tuesday.   8

           c.   The men unloaded 27 of them before noon.   8

           d.   The phone is being installed on 5th May.   8

           e.   They applied for it about 36 months ago.   8

Set the left-hand margin stop at 15, and the line-space lever for single-line spacing.

DRILL 59

They may make the idle men lend a hand to cut the corn.   11

DRILL 60

     We are sorry to complain about the typewriter we   10
bought from you recently. It has given little   19
satisfaction since we have had it, and the mechanic   29
has called in four times already to repair it. We   39
are sending it back to you today, and trust you will   49
replace it with a new one.   54

DRILL 104 (a)

One of your faults may be that you often type an R in the place of a T and vice versa. Practise words such as: roots, trust, dirty, tarts, track, strut, string, turret and porter. **(35 words)**

DRILL 104 (b)

Last week we returned to you several pairs of defective gloves. This week we have had further complaints and are returning fifteen pairs. In view of this we shall, in future, place our order elsewhere. **(35 words)**

DRILL 105 (a)

Punctuation marks should be struck lightly, otherwise they pierce the paper. Capital letters should be struck sharply, and the shift key held down while they are struck. If this key is lifted prematurely the letters will appear out of alignment. **(40 words)**

DRILL 105 (b)

Please send me one of the bookcases with three shelved as advertised in today's press. Because the shelves are adjustable the design will be very suitable for my extra large volumes. I enclose cheque for forty pounds, which includes carriage. **(40 words)**

DRILL 106 (a)

When erasing an incorrect word and replacing it by another word of one letter less, leave an extra half space before typing in the correct word, but leave half a space instead of a whole one before typing in a word containing one extra letter. **(45 words)**

DRILL 106 (b)

Everyone should become familiar with the marking on electric plugs for household use. All plugs are fitted with brown 'live' wires, blue 'neutral' ones, and with green and yellow striped ones for 'earth'. These are each marked with their respective initials, L, N and E. **(45 words)**

DRILL 107

There are a number of definite rules for the typist to observe in the display of letters, but, apart from these, a certain amount is left to her own judgement. She should, for instance, see that work she types is correctly placed to fit in with the firm's letter heading. **(50 words)**

Set the left-hand margin stop at 28, and the line-space lever for single-line spacing.

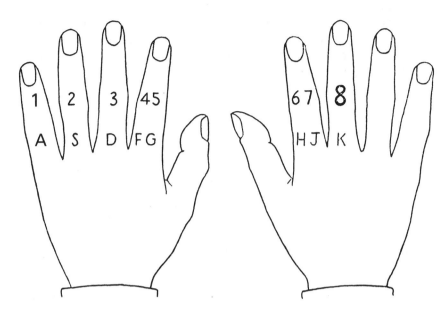

DRILL 61 a. She had to pay the carriage on 78 cases.   8

b. Postage was refunded on 18 damaged ones.   8

c. Each case contains 84 typewriting books.   8

d. I use 1,123 reams of A4 paper each year.   8

e. The typist has typed about 56 envelopes.   8

Set the left-hand margin stop at 15, and the line-space lever for single-line spacing.

DRILL 62

The six men got pay for the work they did for the firm.   11

DRILL 63

Packaging and bottling have changed since Britain   10
adopted the European systems of currency, weights and   21
measures. Items are counted in tens instead of dozens,   32
weight in grams in the place of pounds, the unit of   42
length is the metre and the litre has largely ousted   53
the pint.   55

Set the left-hand margin stop at 30, and the line-space lever for single-line spacing.

In the second line a *colon* is used for the first time. Remember to depress the left shift key before striking the colon, which is above the semicolon.

The position of the fractions differs with the make of machine. Notice the position of the fractions on your machine, and use the appropriate finger in the following sentences:-

DRILL 100 a.   The box measured $5\frac{1}{2}$ x $4\frac{1}{4}$ x $3\frac{1}{4}$.   6

b.   Add $\frac{1}{8}$, $\frac{3}{8}$ and $\frac{5}{8}$: the sum is $1\frac{1}{8}$.   6

c.   A figure $4\frac{1}{2}$ by $4\frac{1}{2}$ is a square.   6

d.   The bookshelf was $24\frac{7}{8}$" by $8\frac{3}{4}$".   6

e.   His niece had $\frac{3}{8}$ of his estate.   6

Set the left-hand margin stop at 15, and the line-space lever for single-line spacing.

The following paragraphs are counted in *standard* words (rather than 5-stroke words). Try to finish each paragraph, accurately, in one minute.

DRILL 101 (a)

    These passages should be attempted when you have a
fair chance of finishing each of them in one minute
accurately. **(20 words)**

DRILL 101 (b)

    When addressing envelopes remember to type the postal
code after the place name, as this facilitates
correct and punctual delivery. **(20 words)**

DRILL 102 (a)

    Now that you have finished all the exercises dealing
with the mastery of the keyboard, you should be able
to type at a fair speed. **(25 words)**

DRILL 102 (b)

    When dividing words at line-endings certain rules must
be applied. Never divide a word of one syllable or
words beginning with a capital letter. **(25 words)**

DRILL 103 (a)

    Do some speed practice for a few minutes every day until
you can type at a really high rate. A high rate means
seventy, eighty or ninety words a minute. **(30 words)**

DRILL 103 (b)

    We ordered a hundred textbooks a month ago but have still
not received them. We need them for the new term and
would be grateful if you could forward them. **(30 words)**

Set the left-hand margin stop at 28, and the line-space lever for single-line spacing.

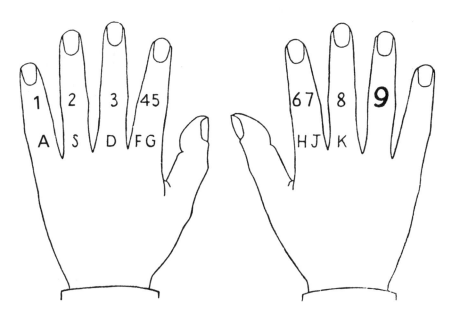

DRILL 64 a. A lease is sometimes taken for 99 years.   8

          b. Leases may also be bought for 999 years.   8

          c. About 14 houses out of 38 need painting.   8

          d. They have started to decorate 56 others.   8

          e. Of 27 erected, 19 were let very quickly.   8

Set the left-hand margin stop at 15, and the line-space lever for single-line spacing.

DRILL 65

A fox robbed the man of the ducks he kept by the lake.   11

DRILL 66

    Many people say that they cannot afford a holiday   10
but it is surprising how much can be saved for a short   21
break each year, by looking after the odd pennies. So   32
many of these odd pennies are wasted during each year by   43
buying carelessly, or by buying articles which are not   52
really needed and are seldom used.   61

Set the left-hand margin stop at 28, and the line-space lever for single-line spacing.

When used as a dash, the hyphen *must have a space before and after it.*

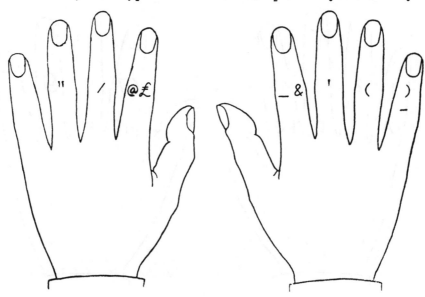

DRILL 97   a.   I am afraid I - er - really do not know.   8

            b.   Go to the shop for the butter - quickly.   8

            c.   It is guaranteed pure - no preservative.   8

            d.   The eggs - two boxes - have not arrived.   8

            e.   It takes five days - no less - to do it.   8

Set the left-hand margin stop at 15, and the line-space lever for single-line spacing.

DRILL 98

When can you deliver the machines we ordered a week ago?   11

DRILL 99

      The dash, as printed, has no special character on   10
the typewriter, and it cannot be reproduced in the same   21
way as in print. Because of this the hyphen is used,   32
but it is essential to distinguish between the use of   43
the hyphen to separate two linked words or syllables and   54
the use of the dash to separate two phrases. The hyphen   65
has no space before or after it if it is used as a   75
hyphen, but a space before and after it when it is used   86
to represent the dash.   90

31

Set the left-hand margin stop at 28, and the line-space lever for single-line spacing.

Use the capital "O" for the *figure nought* if your machine is not fitted with a special key for this character.

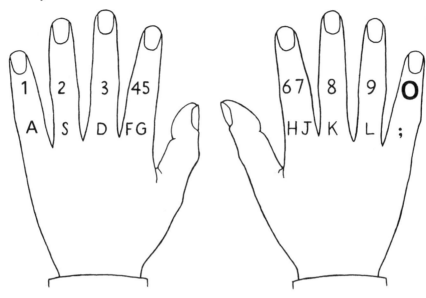

DRILL 67   a.   10 x 10 makes 100 and 90 x 10 makes 900.   8

b.   We ordered 40 kilos of sugar on Tuesday.   8

c.   Rain fell very heavily here for 13 days.   8

d.   1408, 1752 and 1976 were all leap years.   8

e.   The manager may be away until 2nd March.   8

Set the left-hand margin stop at 15, and the line-space lever for single-line spacing.

DRILL 68

The bike he owns is rusty, but he uses it for work.   10

DRILL 69

We understand that you wish to purchase a small   10
car, and we have pleasure in sending you our fully   20
illustrated catalogue containing descriptions of all   31
our latest models for the coming season. Our cars   41
are highly recommended for hard wear and reliability   52
and they compare very favourably with other cars of   62
the type you require.   65

Set the left-hand margin stop at 28, and the line-space lever for single-line spacing.

The two new characters are called the *brackets* or *parentheses*. When typing words in brackets there is no space after the initial bracket or before a final one.

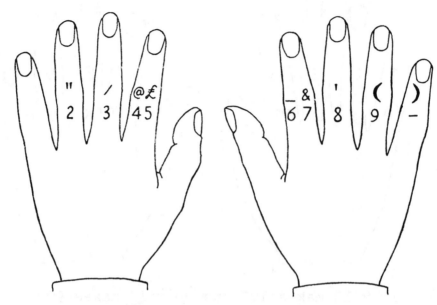

DRILL 94 a. Come and see me at my office (Room 109).   8

          b. She put in two advertisements (prepaid).   8

          c. His father left him £80 (eighty pounds).   8

          d. He was employed by Stags (Builders) Ltd.   8

          e. It is never too late to mend. (Proverb).   8

Set the left-hand margin stop at 15, and the line-space lever for single-line spacing.

DRILL 95

   Our illustrated catalogue of cameras is now in the post.   11

DRILL 96

        If you wish to get a really good post with a good   10
   salary, you should study hard every day to increase your   21
   speeds in the commercial skills. Some people say that   32
   very high speeds are not needed in an office, but, if   43
   your speeds are higher than those you use generally, you   54
   will have the full confidence of always being able to   65
   take down easily anything that may be dictated to you   76
   in shorthand, and transcribe it quickly on the typewriter. 87

Set the left-hand margin stop at 28, and the line-space lever for single-line spacing.

Use the shift key for all the signs above the figures.

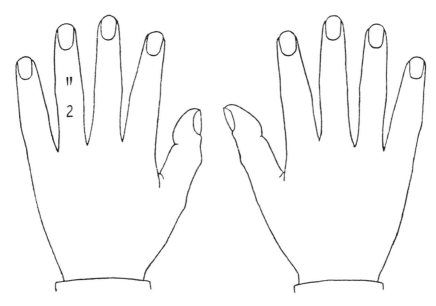

DRILL 70 a. The "Fortune" club has about 50 members.   8

          b. Do you want to be a good "touch" typist?   8

          c. We have read the poem "Under Milk Wood".   8

          d. "I will phone in the morning," said Tom.   8

          e. J. Jones, M.D., "Dawn", Fox Avenue, Ely.   8

Set the left-hand margin stop at 15, and the line-space lever for single-line spacing.

DRILL 71

    Six metres of thick rope were enough for the small job.   11

DRILL 72

        After all punctuation at the end of a sentence,   10
    leave two spaces; but after the punctuation within a   21
    sentence one space only is necessary. When an indented   32
    paragraph is typed, the first line should be indented   43
    five spaces, and the use of the tabulator stop for this   54
    saves the time taken to depress the space bar five   64
    times.   65

Set the left-hand margin stop at 28, and the line-space lever for single-line spacing.

This new sign is called the *hyphen*. Do *not* use the shift key when striking the hyphen.

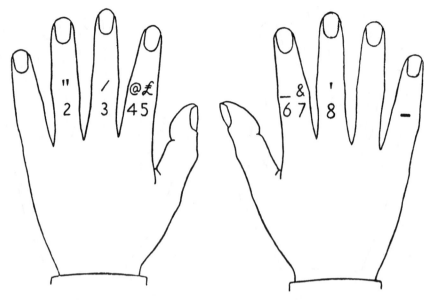

DRILL 91   a.   These four black shirts cost £9.25 each.   8

              b.   The men used six-inch nails for the job.   8

              c.   Sixty-eight soldiers died in the battle.   8

              d.   Capt. J. Bancroft-Browning, V.C., D.S.O.   8

              e.   I wish to purchase a second-hand guitar.   8

Set the left-hand margin stop at 15, and the line-space lever for single-line spacing.

DRILL 92

    The enclosed form will give you the details you need.   11

DRILL 93

          Notice the use of the hyphen in the above sen-   9
tences, and remember that, when using a hyphen to link   20
syllables or words, you do not leave a space before or   31
after it. Notice also that the numbers sixty and eight   42
are linked by a hyphen, as are all the compound numbers   53
from twenty-one to ninety-nine. When cheques are hand-   64
written the hyphen should replace the decimal point in   75
amounts over one pound.   80

Set the left-hand margin stop at 28, and the line-space lever for single-line spacing.

The new sign on the diagram below is called the *solidus*. It is used in instances such as those in the sentences below.

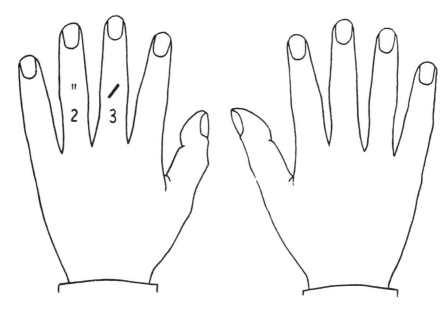

DRILL 73   a.   The return fare, 2nd class, cost me 52p.   8

           b.   His letter, ref. MP/789, was dealt with.   8

           c.   His/her name must be signed on the form.   8

           d.   The boxes of toffees were priced at 67p.   8

           e.   He is not liable for loss and/or damage.   8

Set the left-hand margin stop at 15, and the line-space lever for single-line spacing.

DRILL 74

    We are moving to our new factory at the above address.   11

DRILL 75

        A great number of people, especially men, fill in   10
    the football pools each week in the hope of gaining a   21
    large sum of money in an easy way. They study the   31
    different teams and assess their worth, and then they   42
    forecast which team in each game will win or lose. Some   53
    people are lucky and win a few pounds, but the majority   64
    pay their stakes to no purpose.   70

Set the left-hand margin stop at 28, and the line-space lever for single-line spacing.

The character over the figure eight is called the *apostrophe*. Notice its use in the sentences given below.

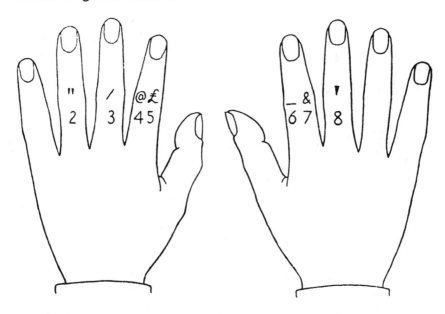

DRILL 88   a.   The lady's handbag and gloves were blue.   8

           b.   The ladies' shoes are not well repaired.   8

           c.   What dreadful weather we have had today.   8

           d.   "It's too much to pay," said Ann to Tom.   8

           e.   Their damaged car was lying on its side.   8

Set the left-hand margin stop at 15, and the line-space lever to single-line spacing.

DRILL 89

    Please complete the enclosed form, and return it to me.   11

DRILL 90

        A combination character is one which is made up   10
of two other characters on the keyboard. There are a   21
number of them, but here is one as an example. Type a   32
full stop, back space once, and then strike the   41
apostrophe. The result obtained will be an exclamation   53
mark. Few machines have on them a key for this mark,   63
and so the character is usually typed in this way.   73

Set the left-hand margin stop at 28, and the line-space lever for single-line
spacing.

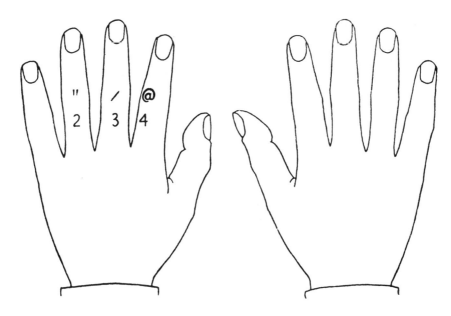

DRILL 76 a. Please forward 24 traycloths @ 89p each.   8

          b. We bought 350 sherry glasses @ 75p each.   8

          c. He charged for 7 km @ 45p per kilometre.   8

          d. The price on the invoice is 6 @ 9p each.   8

          e. The piping cord is priced @ 10p a metre.   8

Set the left-hand margin stop at 15, and the line-space lever for single-line
spacing.

DRILL 77

    Go to the farm at the end of the lane for the butter.   11

DRILL 78

        This new sign is used by typists mainly for lists   10
    of items on an invoice. When lists are typed, the signs 21
    should appear directly under each other, and the amounts 32
    and prices of the goods should also appear in straight   43
    columns with the decimal points under each other. Use   54
    inverted commas for ditto marks to avoid repetition of   65
    the same words in a list.   70

Set the left-hand margin stop at 28, and the line-space lever for single-line
spacing.

The "&" is called the *ampersand*. It is a sign for the word "and". It is
normally used only in sentences such as those given below.

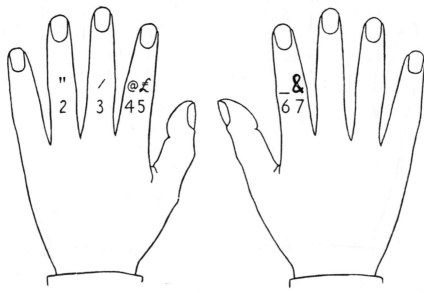

DRILL 85 a. A. Sim & Sons, Bridgend, Looe, PL13 2AD.   8

b. Tod & Bow Ltd., Ringway, Leeds, LS6 2AH.   8

c. Jenkinson & Co. is a very reliable firm.   8

d. Nos. 23, 45, 67, & 89 should be omitted.   8

e. Type Exercises 119 & 225 very carefully.   8

Set the left-hand margin stop at 15, and the line-space lever for single-line
spacing.

DRILL 86

Please let me have the price lists as soon as possible.   11

DRILL 87

The margin stops on the typewriter should always   10
be set before a piece of work is started. When this   21
has been done, a bell will ring to warn the typist that   32
she is approaching the end of the line. After the bell   43
rings, five or six letters may be typed before the   53
carriage is returned for another line. A good typist   64
does not look up at the end of each line.   72

Set the left-hand margin stop at 28, and the line-space lever for single-line
spacing.

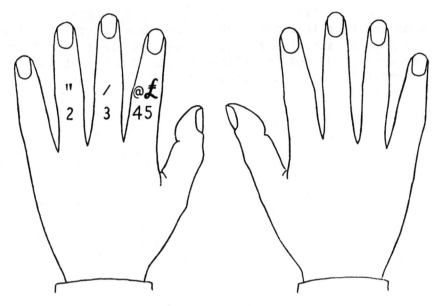

DRILL 79 a. Each man in the firm had a bonus of £60.   8

          b. His account has reached the sum of £427.   8

          c. Has he paid the £3 that he owes you yet?   8

          d. He had to pay £5 for driving so quickly.   8

          e. The price was raised from £10 to £12.85.   8

Set the left-hand margin stop at 15, and the line-space lever for single-line
spacing.

DRILL 80

    If she is paid to do this work, she should do it well.   11

DRILL 81

        Most people have the wish to travel at some time   10
    in their lives. Some do not fulfil this desire because   21
    they cannot decide where to go. If you wish to spend a   32
    holiday abroad, go to an agency in your town where you   43
    will be given all the information you need about an   53
    interesting trip on the Continent. The agent will also   64
    book a room in an hotel for you.   70

Set the left-hand margin stop at 28, and the line-space lever for single-line spacing.

   The character above the figure six is called the *underscore*. It is used to underline words and to rule lines. When words are underlined, the key for the underscore must be struck the exact number of times that there are letters in the word or words. Do *not* underline the punctuation at the end of the line or heading. When returning the carriage to the first letter of the word to be underlined, *do not turn up a line space.*

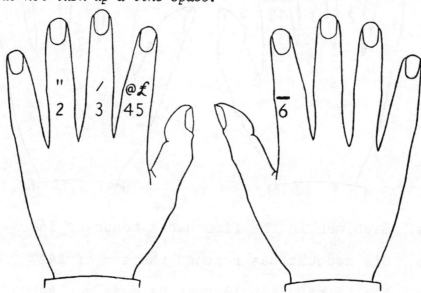

DRILL 82   a.   Please tabulate this <u>exactly</u> as written.   8

           b.   I will meet you all <u>outside</u> the theatre.   8

           c.   <u>N.B.</u>   Delete passages underlined in red.   8

           d.   The women saw the notice "Do Not Smoke".   8

           e.   <u>For the attention of Mr. John Sanderson.</u>   8

Set the left-hand margin stop at 15, and the line-space lever for single-line spacing.

DRILL 83

   The women did the work very quickly with their six mops.   11

DRILL 84

        The underscore, the character over the figure six,   10
   forms a straight line when typed continuously, and is   21
   therefore used to underline words or sentences to   31
   emphasize them. On an electric machine this key can be   42
   held down to produce the line required, and does not   53
   have to be struck as on a manual typewriter. The key   63
   repeats the character automatically.   70

TEACHERS' SUPPLEMENT

Introduction

The aim of this book is the same as that of all other keyboard-training books - to teach the beginner to type accurately and quickly in the shortest possible time. The method used to achieve this aim is, however, very different - the students type complete sentences in the first lesson, and type them as fast as they can.

The drills in this book can be adapted for use in any school, for any age group, and for any length of lesson. It is essential, however, that the teacher should use the book in the way in which it is designed to be used, and for this reason very full notes are given and the first lesson is described in detail.

The First Lesson

Before the first lesson begins, the teacher should insert the paper in each machine, setting the left-hand margin stop at 30, and the line-space lever for single-line spacing. The carriage should be moved to the beginning of the line. This means that the students can begin work immediately they enter the classroom, and that no time is wasted at the beginning of the first lesson. If the room is not available before the lesson starts, it is often possible to arrange with the teacher using the room during the previous lesson for her students to do this. Whatever the arrangements made, it is essential that no time should be wasted. Once the class has assembled, work should begin.

The position of the fingers on the home keys and the use of the right-hand thumb for the space bar should be taught first. Students may then type ASDFG space ;LKJH space three times each on one line, to acquire correct striking of the keys. Then, helped by the teacher, the students memorize the position of the letters shown on the diagram on page 1. The simplest way of doing this is for the students - at first with the help of the teacher, and then on their own - to repeat aloud the letters ED RF TG YH UJ IK, making the necessary finger movements at the same time without actually striking the keys. Once the teacher is sure that the students are familiar with the position of these letters and with the necessary finger movements, she should, if a demonstration machine is available, show the class how the first sentence on page 1 is typed. This demonstration will show the students how to sit at the machine, and where to place the machine in relation to the position of the arms and hands. Very few set rules concerning the position of the typist at her desk should be taught. The ideal position depends upon so many things: the height of the desk; the height of the student; and the length of the student's arms. In the course of the lesson, any minor faults can be corrected. Such advice as "If you sit a little farther from the machine, you will be able to type more quickly"; "If you lift your wrists slightly, your speed will increase"; has been found to be sufficient. The students should be encouraged to make them-selves as comfortable as possible, and to adjust their chairs to the height

Sample of One Lesson's Work

The type on this page is called 'pica'. If your machine has what is called 'elite' type, the letters will appear smaller than in the examples given here.

```
                    tey tired the kire there

                    t ey tierd the kite there

                    they tried the kite there

          "/"       they tried the kite there
                    they tried the kite there
          S.12      they tred

                    the tried the the there
                    they tried the kitr tere
          S.16      they tried the kite there
                    the

                    they tried the kite there
                    they tried the kite there
          S.17      th tried the kite there
                    the they

                    they tried the kite there
                    they tried te dite there
          S.18      theyd tried the kite there
                    they the lite h

                    they tried the kite there
                    they tried the lite there
          S.20      they tried the kite here
                    they treid the kite there

                    they tried the kiw there
                    they tried the kite there
          S.24      they tried the kite there
                    they tried the kite ther
                    they tried the sidt

                    they tried the kite there
          "O"       they tried the kite there
                    they tried the kite there
          S.18      they tried the ki
```

they find most suitable. If necessary, in classes where adjustable chairs are not available, blocks of wood can sometimes be used to raise the desks, and footrests can be improvised.

After the typing of the first sentence has been demonstrated, the students type this sentence once on their own. When they have done this, the teacher shows them how to return the carriage for the second line, and also how to use the carriage-release lever, and then allows them to practise returning the carriage once or twice. (The carriage should be returned at the end of each sentence, however short the sentence may be. The students thus gain practice from the beginning in returning the carriage quickly - this is essential if they are to become good typists.)

After the students have been shown how to return the carriage, they once again repeat aloud the letters on the diagram on page 1, at the same time repeating the finger movements. The first sentence is then typed again, the carriage returned, and the letters on the diagram once more repeated aloud while the finger movements are made. The students should now be sufficiently familiar with the position of the letters to be able to make these finger movements without hesitation. A one-minute accuracy timing is now given during which the students type this first sentence as accurately as they can. They can repeat it as many times as they are able, but the emphasis should be on *accuracy* and not on speed. The carriage is returned at the end of every sentence. At the end of the minute (it should be carefully timed) the students check their work, marking any errors, and noting in the margin the number of mistakes. If there are no mistakes they should write "0" in the margin. The teacher should ask how many students have typed the sentence without making any mistakes, how many have made one mistake, how many two, and so on. If only a few of the students have managed to type accurately during this first accuracy timing, the timing should be repeated once - or more times if necessary (see page 25f for sample of one lesson's work.)

The students should have no difficulty in assessing the speed at which they are typing, as the number of words in each sentence and paragraph in this book is given in bold figures in the right-hand margin. These bold figures indicate the number of words (of five strokes) in the line, or, in the case of paragraphs, the number of words up to that point in the paragraph.

When a reasonable standard of accuracy has been reached, this one-minute timing should be repeated, but this time the students should type as *fast* as they can. Accuracy does not matter during this *speed* timing. Mistakes are ignored and no attempt should be made to correct them. This speed timing should be repeated five or six times, and the teacher should encourage the students to type faster and faster, by asking them repeatedly whether or not they have improved upon their previous highest speeds. The teacher's aim is to force the student to type as quickly as possible, and the speed timing on a particular exercise should be repeated again and again - until the students are no longer improving upon their previous best speeds. The exercises should be typed in single-line spacing, with a double-line space between each one-minute timing. This double-line space will make it much easier for the students to check their results.

teacher should explain to the students that it may be necessary for them to divide words at line-endings, and should give them a few simple rules.

1. A word of one syllable should not be divided.
2. A syllable of one letter should not be left at the end of a line, nor should a syllable of two letters be taken forward to the next line.
3. Words containing double letters are usually divided between the double letters.
4. Words should be divided as far as possible into syllables.

The figures are taught in the same way as the letters of the alphabet, and so are the additional characters. The exercises for the additional characters not only give practice in typing characters, but also show their use. For example, on page 28, the apostrophe is taught. The exercises on this page give examples of the use of the apostrophe - showing especially places where the student is likely to go wrong in using this character - as in the use of "its" and "it's".

When the keyboard has been mastered, the exercises from page 34 onwards can be dealt with in exactly the same way as in the first lesson. Speed tests on page 50-3 will give the students practice in typing longer passages, and by the time they have reached this point they should be able to type at the fifty words a minute required for Advanced Examinations. The 5-stroke words have been included to help both in assessing speed, and also for the benefit of students sitting typewriting examinations for examining bodies where accuracy tests are required.

Speed Timings

THE 5-STROKE METHOD

Count all the letters, spaces and punctuation marks in the passage typed. Divide the result by 5 to give the number of words typed. Then divide by the number of minutes taken. This answer is the speed per minute. This is known as the 5-stroke method.

THE STANDARD METHOD

Count all the words regardless of length (ignoring spaces and punctuation marks) and divide by the number of minutes taken. The answer is the speed per minute. This is called the standard method.

There is a slightly different result. Usually the 5-stroke method gives a higher speed. The reverse would occur only in passages containing a large percentage of words containing four letters or less.

In this book the 5-stroke method has been used, except where the standard method is indicated (standard).

Progress sheets should be prepared in advance, and handed out to the students at this stage. Students can now enter in the margin and on the progress sheet their fastest speeds for this one-minute *speed* timing. If they have typed without making any mistakes during the *accuracy* timing, they may also record their speeds in the second column of the progress sheet. The following is the suggested layout for this progress sheet:-

DATE	SENTENCES			PARAGRAPHS		
	FIRST ACCURACY TIMING	SPEED TIMING	FINAL ACCURACY TIMING	FIRST ACCURACY TIMING	SPEED TIMING	FINAL ACCURACY TIMING

These progress sheets should be completed very carefully, as they will not only give the teacher a very useful record of the students' progress, but they will give the students themselves an incentive to do better in both the speed and accuracy timings. During the accuracy timing speed does not matter, provided that the exercise is typed accurately, and no entries should be made in the second column unless no mistakes have been made during this timing. At first, the students are likely to make an occasional error, but they should become more accurate as the course proceeds.

During the first few lessons, only the first four columns of the progress sheet will be used. At the end of the course, the students should have, in all the columns, a complete record of their progress and of the standard they have reached.

When the speed timings have been repeated five or six times, a final *accuracy* timing is given on this sentence. The work is checked, and the speed and the number of errors entered in the margin. If necessary, an entry is also made on the progress sheet. Already, after only a short time has elapsed in the first lesson, the students can see from this record that they are making progress.

Each sentence (and later on the paragraphs) is dealt with in this way.

Paper insertion is taught directly the first student reaches the end of the first page of typescript. After this, the students should be expected to insert fresh paper into their machines as quickly as possible in the course of their work. The teacher should not wait for students to do this. They will do it much more quickly if they know that they are missing part of their typewriting lesson. Quick paper handling is another essential if they are to become good typists, and the method used in this book is designed to encourage this. Throughout the lesson, no time is wasted. Ten seconds is a sufficient interval between each one-minute timing.

To summarize the work of the first lesson:-

1. Class assembles (paper inserted and machines ready for use).
2. Teacher teaches the position of the keys on page 1.
3. Class repeats letters aloud, making finger movements.
4. Teacher demonstrates typing of first sentence.
5. Students type sentence once.
6. Teacher teaches carriage return and carriage-release lever.
7. Students repeat letters aloud.
8. Students type sentence once.
9. Students repeat letters aloud.
10. Students type sentence for one minute *accurately*, as many times as they can.
11. Students type sentence for one minute *quickly*. This speed timing is repeated seven or eight times.
12. Students type sentence for one minute *accurately*.

Subsequent Lessons

The pattern of all subsequent lessons follows the pattern of the first lesson. As the students progress, the accuracy timings can be increased by one minute at a time, up to five minutes. Ten-minute accuracy tests should be given only when preparing for examinations. It is important to note that the duration of *speed* timings is never increased beyond one minute.

The supplementary exercises in this book have been very carefully compiled to help the student to secure a complete mastery of the keyboard. In the first six pages care has been taken to include sentences containing common combinations of letters and, at the same time, to choose sentences with a variety of subject matter.

When the letters of the keyboard have been mastered, a period of consolidation work follows. At the same time, the subject matter of the exercises is very varied, and includes some points on the theory of typewriting. The students will thus learn some of the theory of typewriting while they are actually producing typewritten work.

The remainder of the theory necessary at this stage should be taught between the speed timings, as it becomes necessary. The use of the space bar is taught before any work is started. The use of the carriage-return lever is taught when the students have typed one sentence. Paper insertion is taught when the first student completes a page of typescript; the shift key when capital letters are first introduced on page 6; the tabulator when paragraph indentations are introduced on page 13.

The most difficult part of the theory to teach is probably the division of words at line-endings, and for this reason some notes are given for the teacher's guidance. It is not necessary for the student to be taught how to divide words at line-endings until page 34 is reached, as, up to that point, all the exercises are reproductions of typewriting and the student has only to follow the line-endings already given. When page 34 is reached, the